50 Keto Desserts Recipes

Table of Contents

INTRODUCTION

The term "keto desserts" sounds like an oxymoron, right up there with colossal shrimp and deafening stillness. After all, isn't the whole point of the keto diet to cut out all sweets? Knowing the fundamentals of how keto works is critical in order to understand what desserts you can and can't have and, more significantly, how to stay on track.

One of the most common flaws we notice in the keto diet is approaching it from the wrong perspective. So many people are hoping for a quick cure that may be completed in a few weeks. Perhaps they need to lose 10 pounds for a wedding, reunion or swimming suit season, and they'd like to lose a few pounds for a few months. They don't mind how things go as long as the work gets done.

Crash dieting, which is described as an eating pattern used to lose weight that isn't sustainable, is common. Keto is a long-term lifestyle decision, and we encourage everyone who attempts the diet to embrace this mindset. It doesn't mean you're committing to eating this way for the rest of your life; it only means you could if you wanted to. You'll always be looking for balance if you eat a keto diet. When cravings strike and the pounds begin to creep back on, eating sensibly keeps you out of trouble.

This dessert cookbook contains all the recipes which are the best substitute for those unhealthy dishes which are not best to eat. Eating a diet high in processed and refined carbohydrates may alter the balance of gut bacteria and cause blood sugar to rise and fall significantly, both of which can adversely affect skin health. These low carb desserts could reduce acne symptoms in some people and helps to maintain a sugar level.

KETO CLASSIC CINNAMON SUGAR DONUT

Prep Time: 10 Minutes

Cook Time: 15 Minutes

Serves: 12

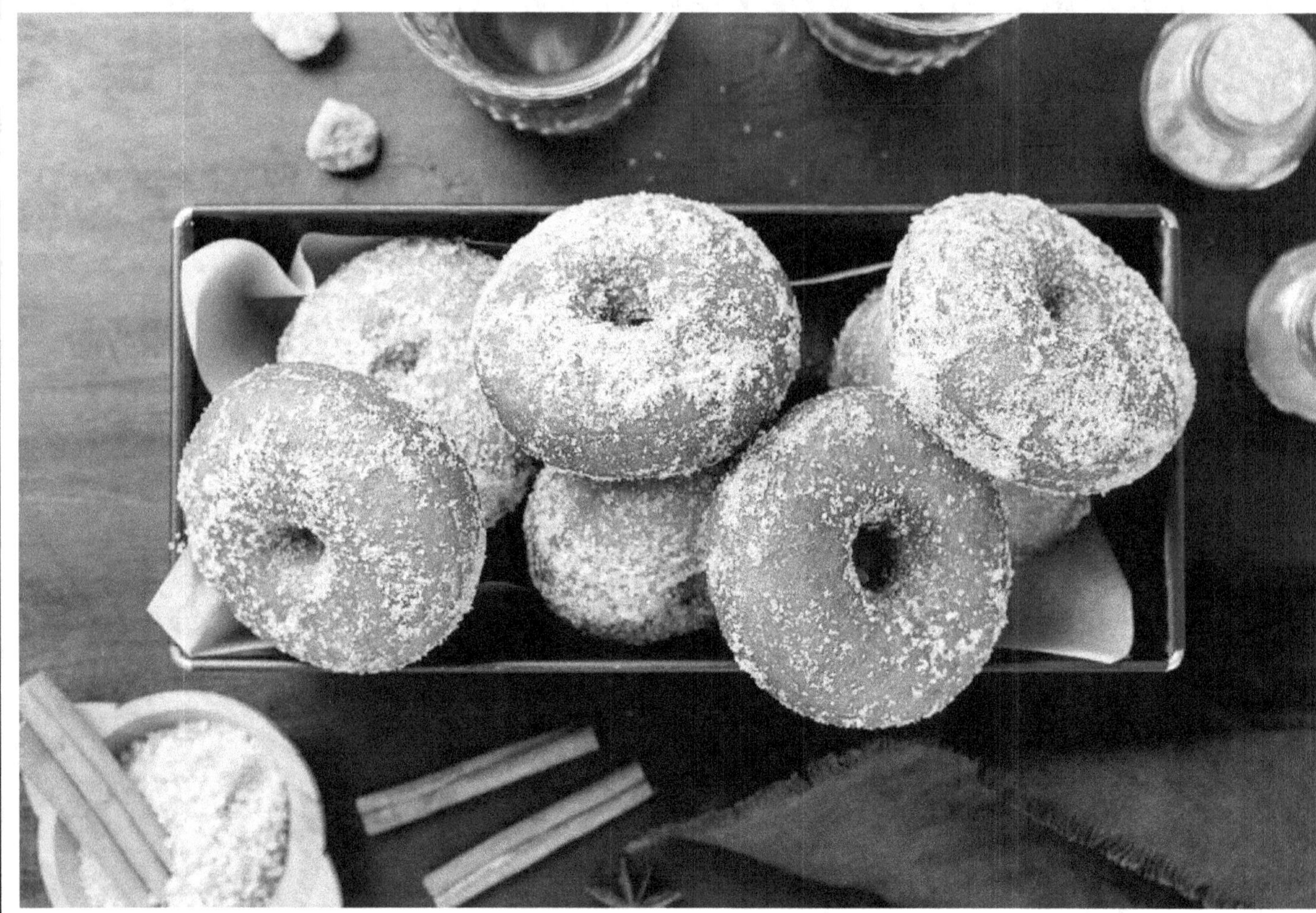

Low-carb doughnuts that are soft and pillowy are great for breakfast, midday snacking, or whenever you're craving a classic cinnamon sugar donut from the fair. Best of all, this delectable dish is simple to prepare and does not require the use of a mixer. Paleo, sugar-free, grain-free, and gluten-free are all terms used to describe a diet that is free of grains, sugar.

Nutrition

Calories: 86 | Protein: 2g | Fat: 8g | Saturated Fat: 2g | Carbohydrates: 2g

Ingredients

- 1/4 cup granulated monk fruit sweetener
- 1 cup super-fine blanched almond flour
- 2 large eggs room temperature
- 1/4 teaspoon apple cider vinegar
- 1 1/2 teaspoons baking powder
- 1 teaspoon ground cinnamon
- 1/2 teaspoon baking soda
- 1/4 teaspoon xanthan gum
- 2 tablespoons melted ghee
- 1/4 cup unsweetened almond milk
- 1/2 tablespoon coconut flour
- 1 teaspoon vanilla extract
- mini donut pan
- 1/8 fine sea salt

<u>Topping Choices</u>

- For the Cinnamon Sugar Coating:
- 1 1/2 tablespoons melted ghee, or butter if not paleo
- 1 teaspoon ground cinnamon
- 1/4 cup granulated monk fruit
- For the Chocolate Glaze:
- 1 teaspoon powdered monk fruit sweetener
- 2 ounces No dark sugar chocolate, melted
- 1 teaspoon coconut oil, melted

Instructions

1. Whisk together the eggs, almond milk, apple cider vinegar, melted ghee, vanilla, and monk fruit sweetener in a large bowl until smooth and blended.
2. Combine the almond flour, coconut flour, xanthan gum, cinnamon, baking powder, baking soda, and salt in a separate medium mixing bowl. Add the dry ingredients to the wet components in a slow, steady stream, stirring until just mixed.
3. Fill a greased 12 cavity silicone mini donut pan halfway with batter.
4. Bake until golden brown in a 350F preheated oven for twelve to fifteen minutes for tiny or twenty-one to twenty-four for regular-sized.
5. Remove the pan from the oven and set it aside to cool until the donuts are safe to handle.

<u>For the Cinnamon Coating</u>

1. In a small bowl, combine the granulated sweetener and cinnamon while the donuts are baking.
2. Melt the ghee in a separate small heat-safe dish (or butter).
3. Lightly immerse each cooled donut in melted ghee before rolling in the cinnamon/sweetener coating.
4. Continue with the remaining donuts.

<u>For the Chocolate Glaze</u>

1. In a small heat-safe bowl, combine the chopped chocolate and coconut oil and melt in the microwave. Stir in the sweetener until it is fully incorporated.
2. Place the chocolate-coated donuts in the fridge until the chocolate coating has hardened.

SUGAR-FREE CHOCOLATE BARK WITH BACON AND ALMONDS

Prep Time: 20 Minutes

Cook Time: 5 Minutes

Serves: 8

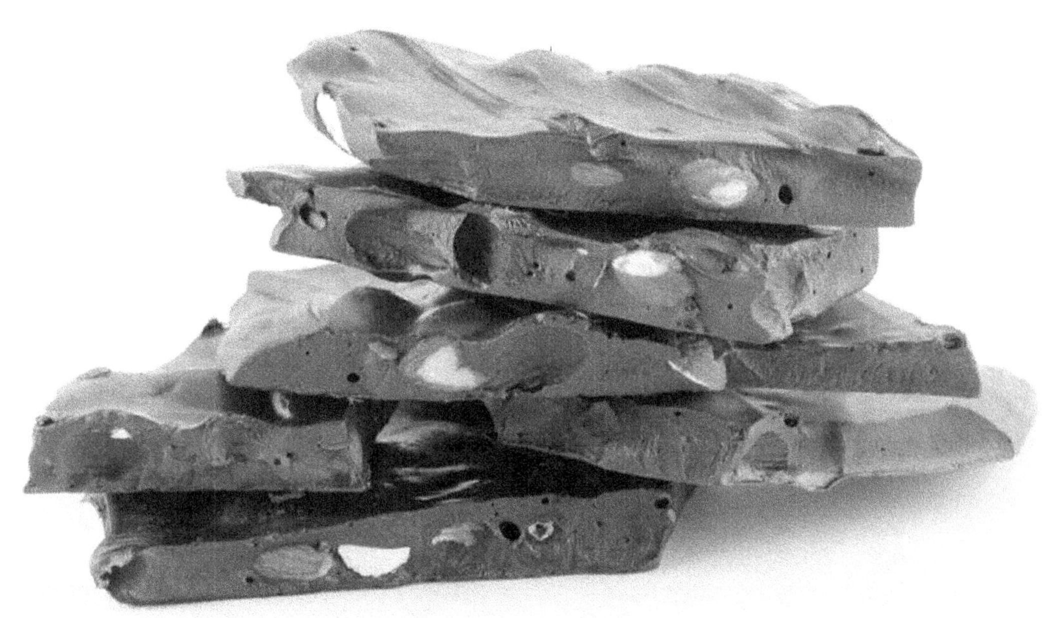

This delectable sugar-free chocolate bark with bacon and almonds is only 3 ingredients and 25 minutes away. There will be no excuses to fall off the low-carb wagon with this low-carb dessert because it is so simple to create.

Nutrition

Calories: 157cal | Fat: 12.8g | Fiber: 7.5g | Protein: 4g | Carbohydrates: 12.7g

Ingredients

- 2 slices bacon cooked and crumbled
- ½ cup Chopped Almonds
- 1 9 oz bag Sugar-free Chocolate Chips

Instructions

1. Microwave the chocolate chips for thirty seconds on high in a microwave-safe bowl, stirring halfway through. Stir after another thirty seconds in the microwave. Stir one more after fifteen seconds in the microwave. When you take it out of the microwave, make sure a few un-melted chocolate chips are left. Then give it one last swirl to make sure it's fully melted.
2. Pour the melted chocolate mixture in a thin layer, about 1/2 inch, on a parchment prepared baking sheet and stir in the chopped almonds.
3. Sprinkle the crumbled bacon over the chocolate and use a spatula to push it in.
4. Break the chocolate into 8 pieces after peeling away the parchment. Refrigerate for at least twenty minutes or until the chocolate has hardened fully. Refrigerate any leftovers.

CHOCOLATE KETO PIE

Prep Time: 4 Hours

Cook Time: 15 Minutes

Serves: 8

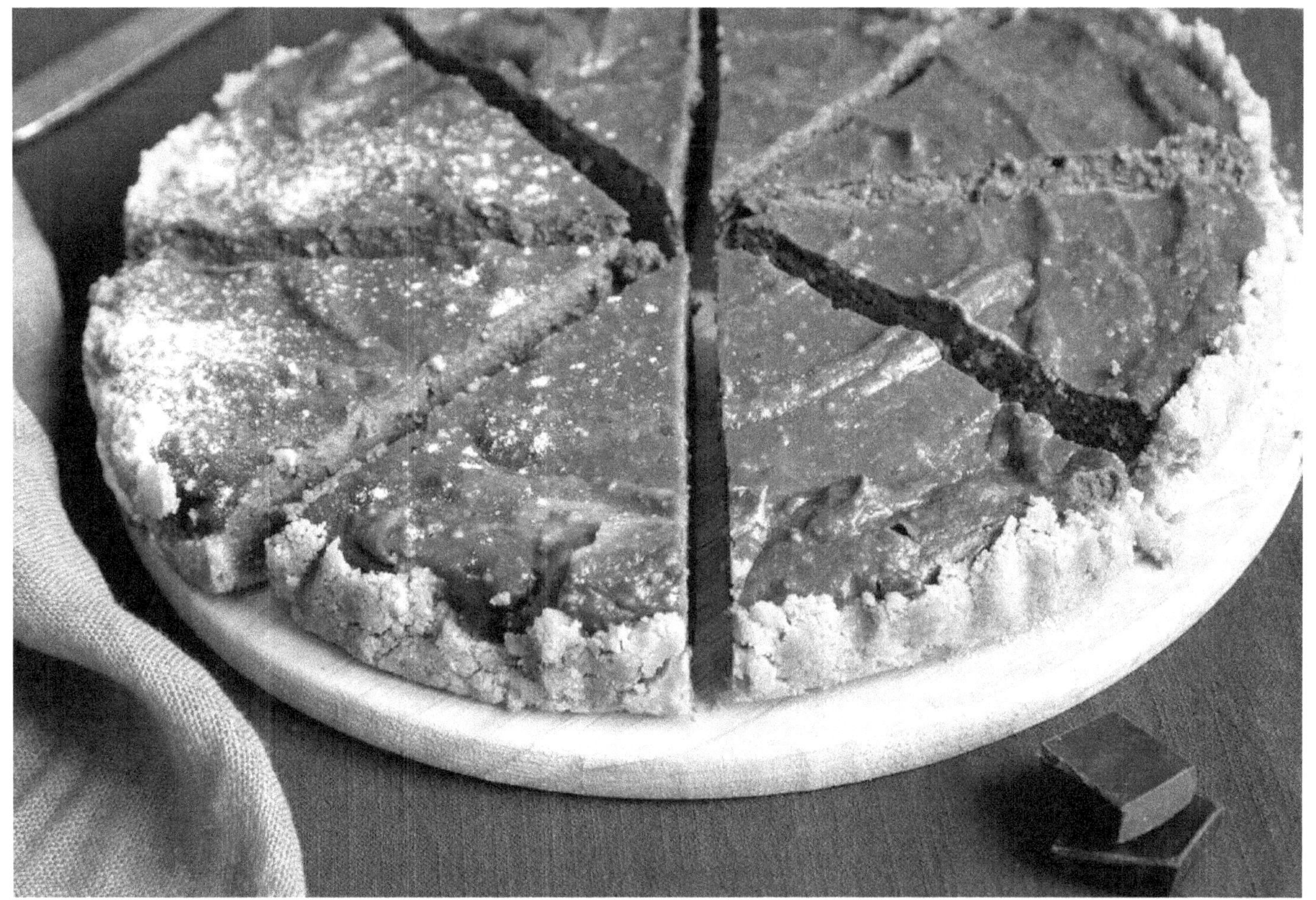

A silky smooth, sugar-free chocolate pudding filling sits atop a melt-in-your-mouth almond flour and butter crust in this Low Carb and Keto pie. This is the ideal holiday treat

Nutrition

Calories: 424kcal | Carbohydrates: 5g | Fiber: 8g | Sugar: 1g | Fat: 38g

Saturated Fat: 12g

Ingredients

- 6 pieces Unsweetened bakers' chocolate, chopped
- 3 Egg yolks
- 1 Almond Flour Pie Crust
- 1 cup Granular Sweetener
- 1 tablespoon Corn starch
- 1 teaspoon Vanilla extract
- 2 teaspoons xanthan gum
- 3 Tablespoons Cocoa Powder
- ¼ teaspoon Kosher salt
- 2 Tablespoons Butter
- 2 cups Unsweetened Almond Milk

Instructions

1. Remove the pie crust from the oven and set it aside to cool.
2. In a medium saucepan, mix together the Swerve, corn starch, xanthan gum, and salt. Next, whisk together the egg yolks, vanilla, almond milk, and chocolate powder. Heat over a medium heat setting.
3. Remove the pan from the heat when the mixture begins to boil and thickens to the consistency of pudding, then whisk in the chopped chocolate and butter until thoroughly melted.
4. Pour the chocolate pudding into the pie crust and set it aside for at least four hours in the refrigerator.
5. Serve with whipped cream on the side.

KETO CHOCOLATE CHIP COOKIES

Prep Time: 10 Minutes

Cook Time: 15 Minutes

Serves: 21

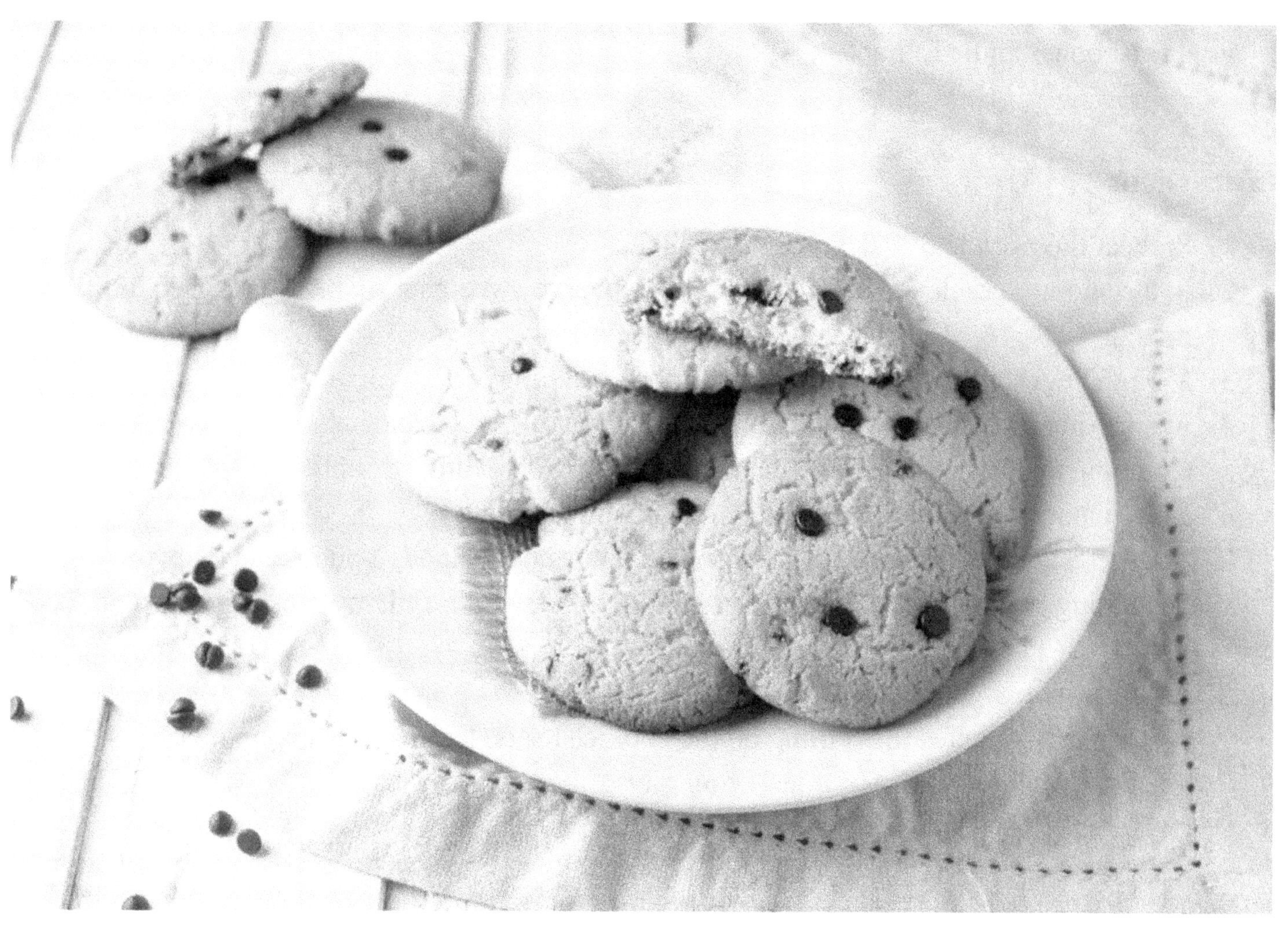

These low-carb, gluten-free keto chocolate chip cookies are simple to make, incredibly delicious, and kid-approved! All you'll need is a single bowl. This recipe calls for almond flour.

Nutrition

Calories: 179kcal | Carbohydrates: 4g | Fat: 17g | Fiber: 2g | Protein: 5g

Ingredients

- 2 Eggs
- 3 cups almond flour
- ½ 9 Ounce Bag Sugar-free Chocolate Chips
- ¾ cup Softened butter or coconut oil
- ½ teaspoon Baking soda
- ⅔ cup Granular Sweetener
- ½ teaspoon Kosher salt
- 2 teaspoon Vanilla Extract

Instructions

1. Preheat the oven to 350 degrees Fahrenheit.
2. In a stand mixer, blend softened butter and swerve sweetener on medium speed until mixed.
3. Mix in 2 eggs and the vanilla extract until everything is well mixed.
4. In a medium mixing bowl, add almond flour, baking soda, and salt.
5. Combine the dry and wet ingredients in a mixing bowl and stir until well blended.
6. Lily's Chocolate Chips should be folded in at this point.
7. Scoop 18-21 cookies onto a baking sheet that has been lined. You may need two, depending on how big your sheets are. Flatten them out a little by pressing down on the top.
8. Bake ten-twelve minutes in the oven
9. Allow thirty minutes for cooling on the cookie sheets. In an airtight container, these will keep soft and delicious for at least four days.

KETO CHEESECAKE FLUFF

Prep Time: 10 Minutes

Cook Time: 0 Minutes

Serves: 6

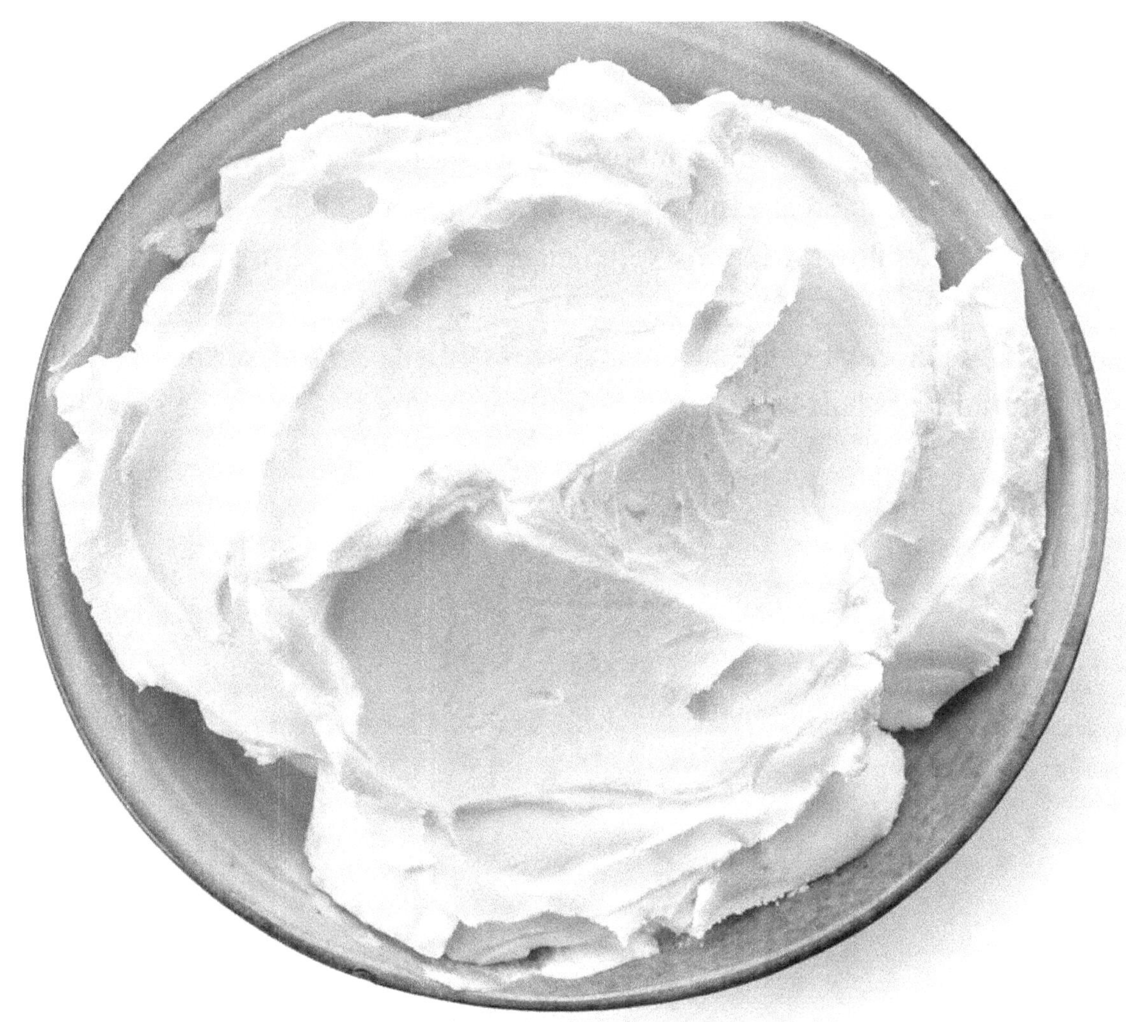

A four-ingredient keto cheesecake fluff that can be stacked with whatever toppings your heart desires! It also has five topping options and four mix-in options for various flavors.

Nutrition

Calories: 258kcal | Carbohydrates: 4g | Fiber: 0g | Sugar: 2g | Saturated Fat: 17g

Protein: 4g | Fat: 27g

Ingredients

- 1 8 ounces Brick of Cream Cheese, Softened
- 1 cup Heavy Whipping Cream
- ½ Cup Granular Sweetener
- Zest of 1 Lemon

Instructions

1. Make the Fluff
2. In a stand mixer, whisk together the heavy cream and the sugar until stiff peaks form. You can alternatively use a hand mixer or a whisk to beat the mixture by hand.
3. Remove the whipped cream and set it aside in a separate bowl.
4. In the stand mixer bowl, whip the softened cream cheese, zest, and sweetener until smooth.
5. Pour the whipped cream into the cream cheese-filled stand mixer bowl. With a spatula, gently stir until it is halfway incorporated. Finish whipping with the stick blender until smooth.
6. Serve with a topping of your choice.

KETO CHOCOLATE CAKE WITH WHIPPED CREAM ICING

Prep Time: 10 Minutes

Cook Time: 25 Minutes

Serves: 9

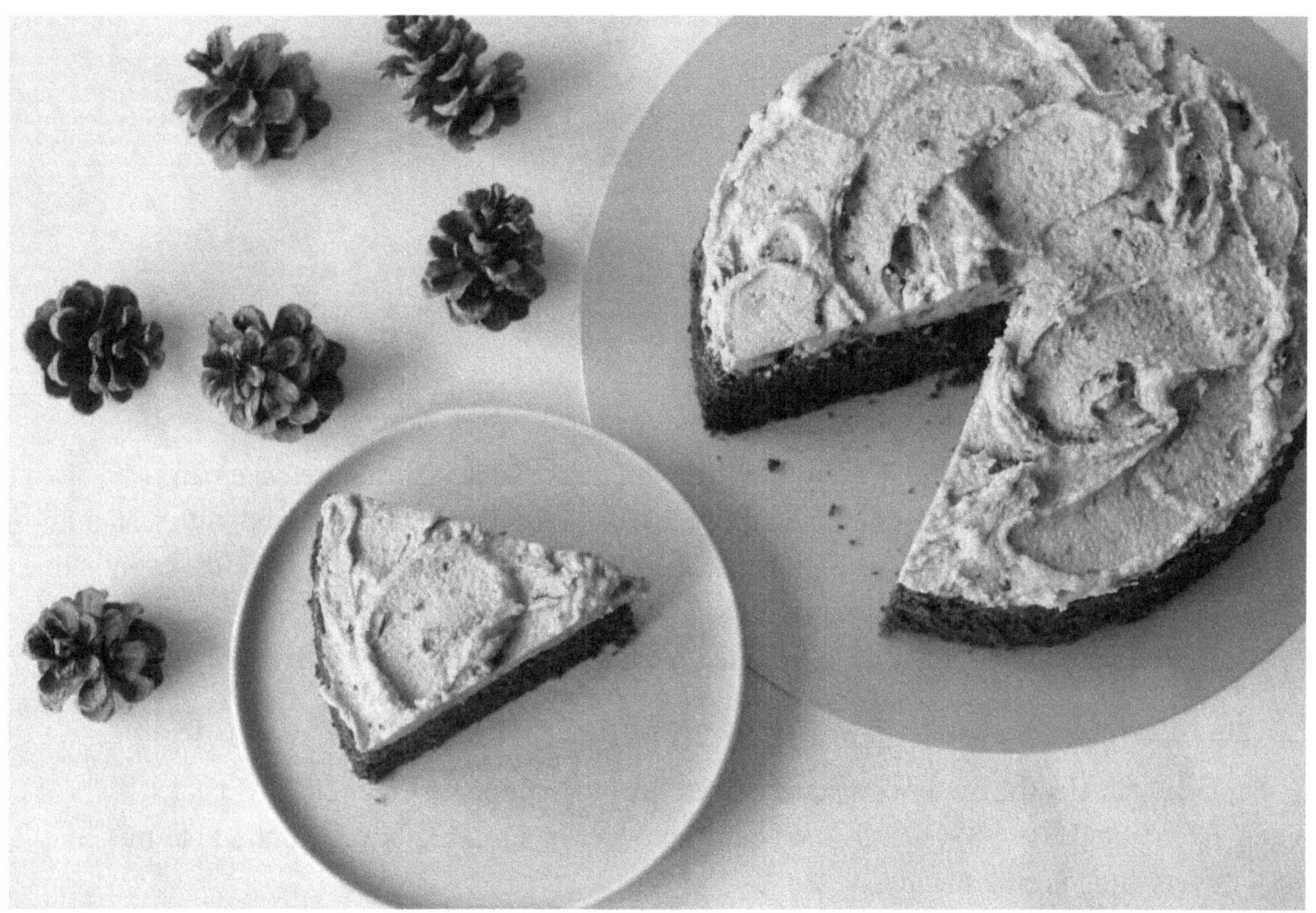

This amazing keto chocolate cake comes together in just one bowl, has the correct cake texture, and the whipped cream topping is just right. This combination will satisfy any chocolate cake cravings you may have.

Nutrition

Calories: 358 | Fat: 33g | Carbohydrates: 11g | Fiber: 6g | Protein: 8g

Ingredients

- 6 Eggs
- 2 teaspoons Baking powder
- ¾ Cup Granular Sweetener
- ⅔ Cup Heavy Whipping Cream
- ½ Cup Melted Butter
- ¾ Cup Coconut flour
- ½ Cup Cocoa powder

Whipped Cream Icing

- ⅓ Cup Sifted Cocoa Powder
- 1 cup Heavy Whipping Cream
- 1 teaspoon Vanilla extract
- ¼ Cup Granular Sweetener

Instructions

1. Preheat the oven to 350 degrees Fahrenheit. Grease an 8-inch square cake pan.
2. In a large mixing bowl, combine all of the cake ingredients and beat well with a stand mixer or an electric mixer. Fill the cake pan halfway with batter and bake for twenty-five minutes, or until the middle springs back when lightly touched.
3. Before icing, remove the cake from the oven and allow it to cool fully.

For the Icing

1. Using an electric mixer or a stand mixer, beat the whipping cream to stiff peaks. Combine the swerve, vanilla, and cocoa powder in a mixing bowl. Continue to mix until everything is well blended.
2. Using the frosting, frost the cake and serve. Any leftovers must be refrigerated.

KETO BROWN BUTTER PRALINES

Prep Time: 5 Minutes

Cook Time: 12 Minutes

Chill Time: 60 Minutes

Serves: 10

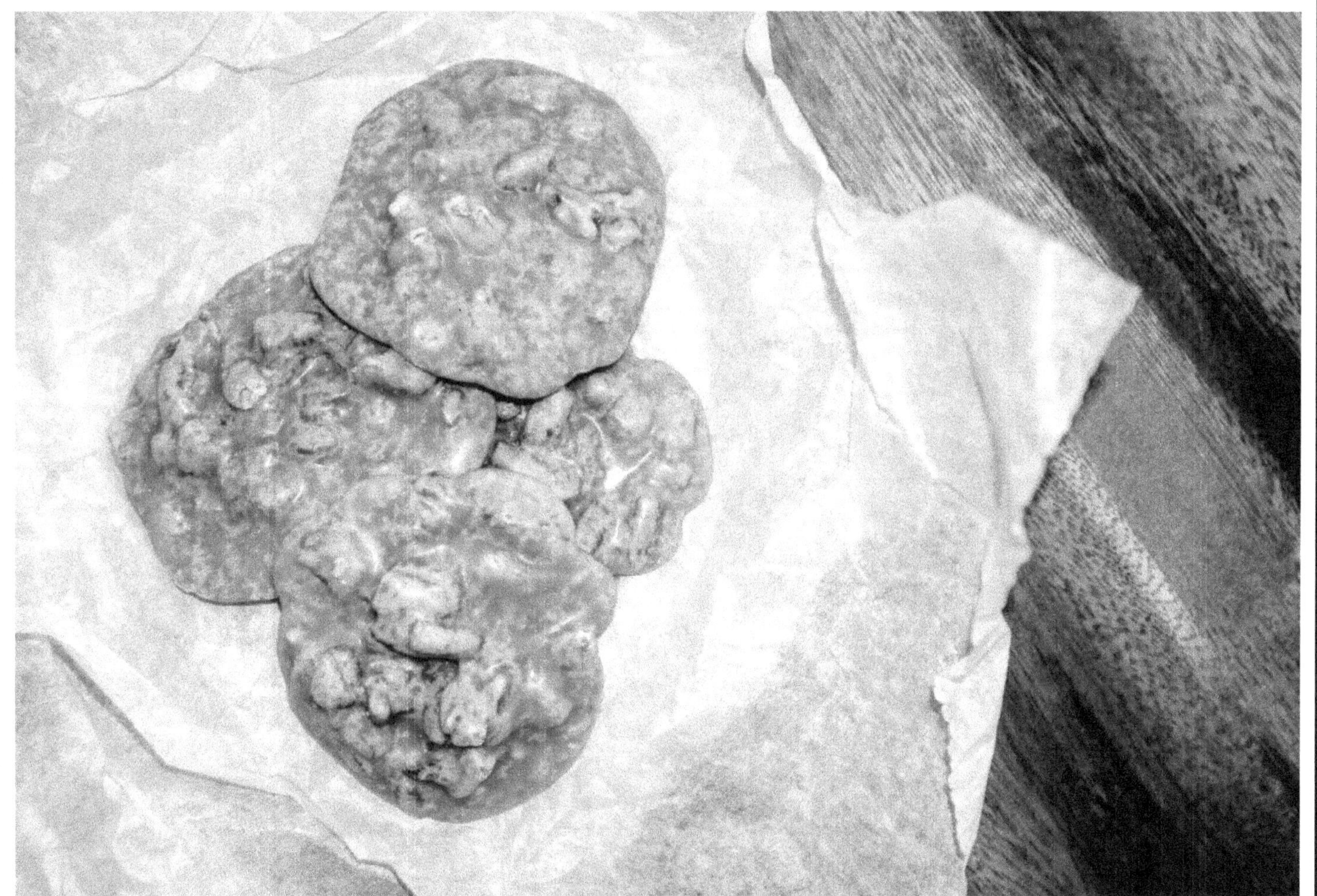

These pecan and cream keto pralines are the ultimate quick holiday dessert. My whole family loves them, and they're only 1 net carb! They firm up in the refrigerator for a couple of hours after a brief cook on the stove. It's that simple.

Nutrition

Calories: 338 | Fat: 36g | Fiber: 2g | Protein: 2g | Carbohydrates: 3g

Ingredients

- ⅔ Cup Granular Sweetener
- ½ teaspoon xanthan gum
- 2 Cups Chopped pecans
- 2 Sticks Salted butter
- ⅔ Cup Heavy Cream
- Maldon sea salt

Instructions

1. Use parchment paper or a silicone baking mat to line a cookie sheet.
2. In a saucepan over medium-high heat, brown the butter, stirring often. This should only take about five minutes. Combine the heavy cream, xanthan gum, and sweetener in a mixing bowl. Turn off the heat.
3. Stir in the nuts and set aside for one hour to firm up, stirring once in a while. The mixture will thicken considerably. Scoop into 10 cookie shapes and place them on the prepared baking sheet. If preferred, sprinkle with Maldon salt. Refrigerate until firm on the baking sheet.
4. Refrigerate until ready to serve in an airtight container.

KETO CHOCOLATE MOUSSE

Prep Time: 10 Minutes

Cook Time: 10 Minutes

Serves: 4

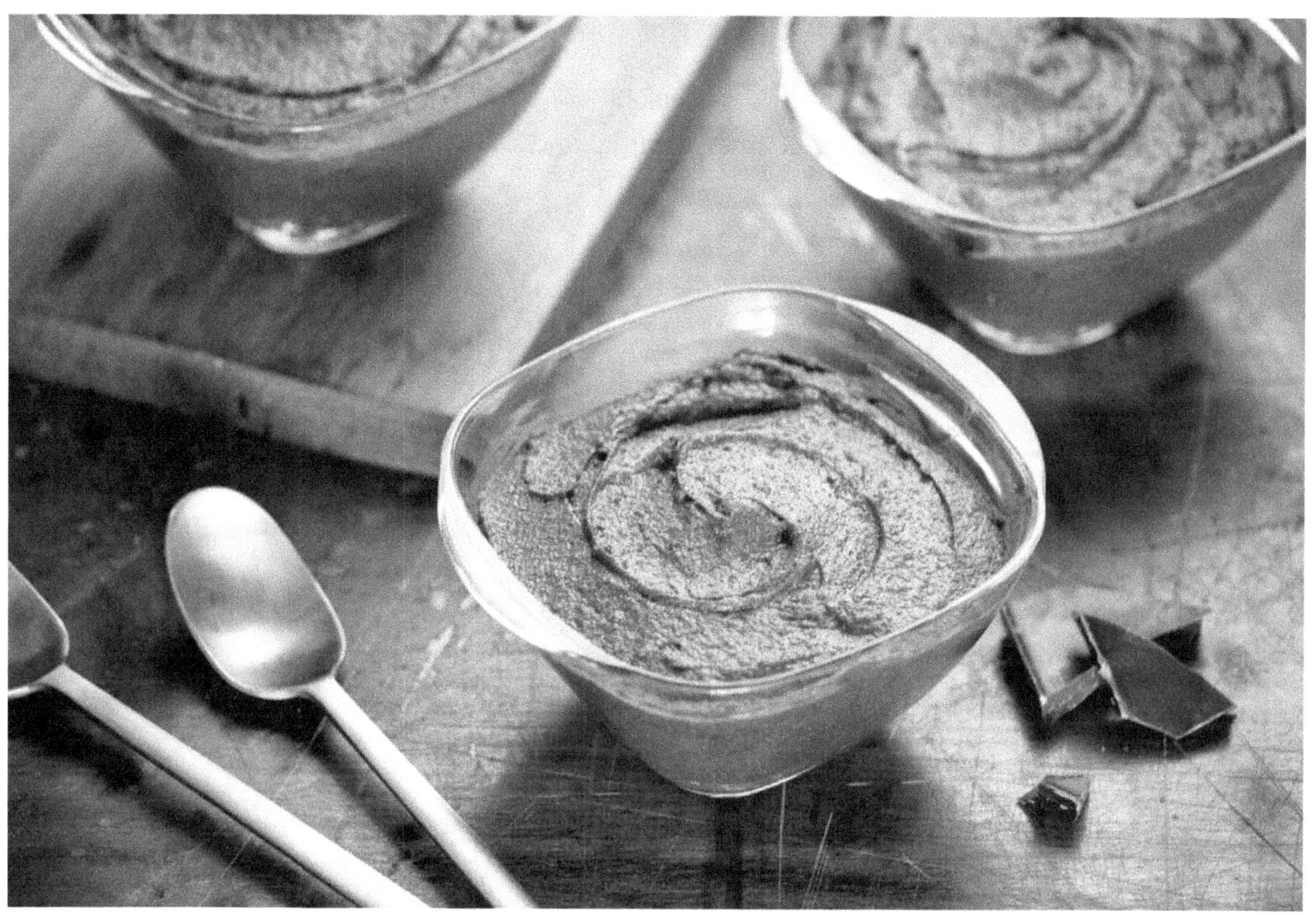

This delectable, low-carb, and keto chocolate mousse is simple to create. Heavy cream, sugar, unsweetened cocoa, and vanilla are the only four ingredients, and no chilling is required

Nutrition

Calories: 218 | Fat: 23g | Fiber: 2g | Protein: 2g | Carbohydrates: 5g

Ingredients

- ¼ cup Unsweetened cocoa powder, sifted
- ¼ cup Powdered Sweetener
- 1 cup Heavy Whipping Cream
- ¼ teaspoon kosher salt
- 1 teaspoon Vanilla extract

Instructions

1. Using a whisk, whip the cream to stiff peaks.
2. Whisk in the cocoa powder, sweetener, vanilla, and salt until everything is well blended.
3. It serves 4 people.

THE BEST KETO CHEESECAKE

Prep Time: 20 Minutes

Cook Time: 50 Minutes

Setting Time: 6-8 Hours

Serves: 12

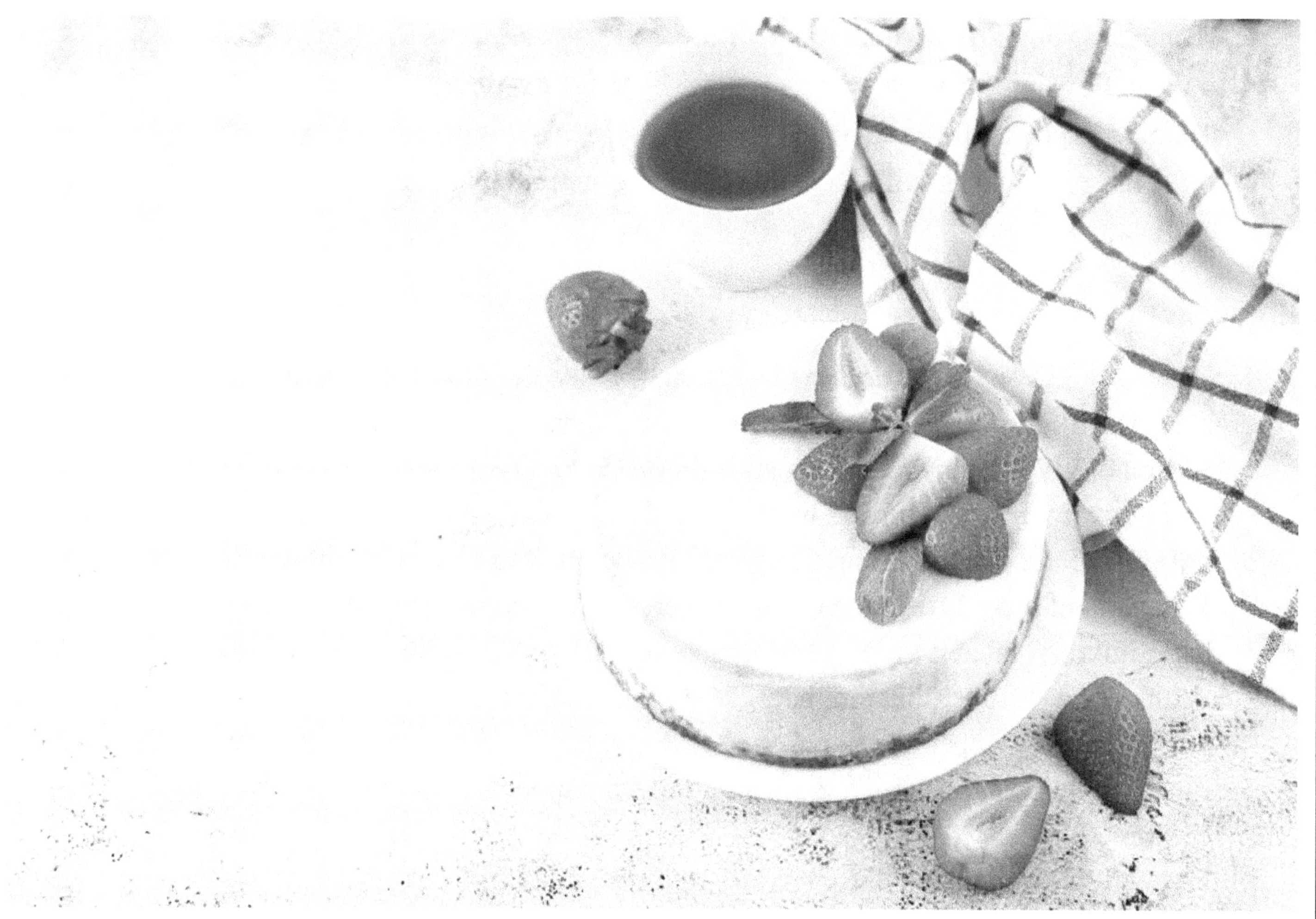

This is the best low-carb and keto cheesecake recipe. "This is the finest cheesecake ever tasted," even the non-keto family exclaimed.

Nutrition

Calories: 600kcal | Carbohydrates: 7g | Saturated Fat: 31g | Fiber: 2g

Protein: 14g | Fat: 54g

Ingredients

<u>For the crust</u>

- 6 tablespoons butter, melted
- ¼ Cup Powdered Sweetener
- 1 ½ Cups almond flour
- 1 teaspoon Cinnamon

<u>For the filling</u>

- 5 Large Eggs room temperature
- 8 Ounces Sour Cream room temperature
- 2 Cups Powdered Sweetener
- 1 tablespoon Vanilla extract
- 6 Packages 8 ounces full fat cream cheese, room temperature

Instructions

1. Preheat the oven to 325 degrees Fahrenheit. Place the rack in the center of the oven. In a medium mixing bowl, combine the dry crust ingredients. Add the butter and stir to combine. Fill a 10-inch x 4-inch springform pan halfway with the crust ingredients and press down with your fingers halfway up the sides. To push the mixture into the bottom of the cup, use a flat-bottomed cup. Allow the crust to chill for twenty minutes.
2. With a hand mixer, whip the room temperature cream cheese until light and fluffy in a large mixing dish. Use the paddle attachment if you're using a stand mixer.
3. With the hand mixer, beat in the sweetener a bit at a time (around 1/3).
4. Add the room temperature eggs one at a time, beating vigorously after each addition.
5. Finally, whisk in the vanilla extract and room temperature sour cream until just combined.
6. Preheat the oven to 350°F. After fifty minutes, double-check. Fill the crust with the cheesecake ingredients and smooth over the top. The top shouldn't be shiny anymore, but the center should still be jiggly.
7. Close the oven door and turn it off. Allow thirty minutes for the cheesecake to cool in the oven. Remove the cheesecake from the oven and run a sharp paring knife between it and the pan to prevent the cake from sticking. Remove the springform but leave it in place. Allow sitting for one hour on the counter.
8. Refrigerate for at least six-eight hours, covered loosely with plastic wrap.

KETO PECAN CRESCENT COOKIES

Prep Time: 45 Minutes

Cook Time: 20 Minutes

Serves: 20

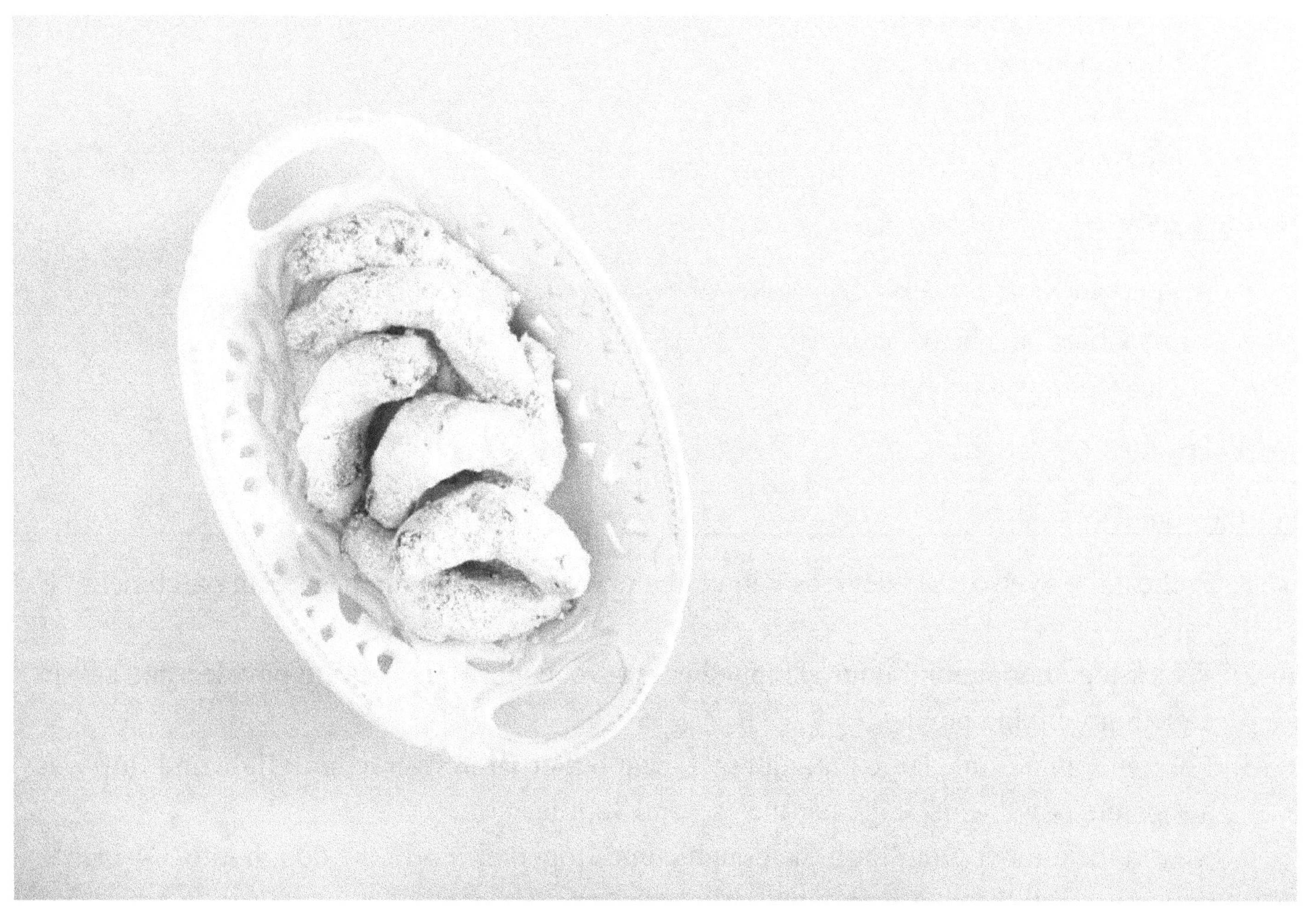

Almond flour is used to make tender pecan crescent pastries. These low-carb cookies are simple to make and tasty. They're perfect for the holidays. They also make delicious snowball cookies! You can eat as much as you like with only 4g total Carbohydrates per serving.

Nutrition

Calories: 168kcal | Carbohydrates: 3.8g | Fat: 15.5g | Fiber: 2g

Protein: 3.5g

Ingredients

<u>Cookies</u>

- 1 large egg
- 2 cups almond flour
- 2 tablespoon coconut flour
- 1/2 teaspoon baking powder
- 1 cup finely chopped pecans
- 1/2 cup butter softened
- 1/2 teaspoon vanilla extract
- 2/3 cup Swerve Brown
- 1/4 teaspoon salt

<u>Vanilla Glaze</u>

- 2/3 cup powdered Swerve Sweetener or powdered erythritol
- 6 to 8 tablespoon heavy cream
- 1/2 teaspoon vanilla extract

Instructions

<u>For the cookies</u>

1. Preheat the oven to 325 degrees Fahrenheit and line two baking pans with parchment paper.
2. Whisk together almond flour, chopped pecans, coconut flour, baking powder, and salt in a medium mixing bowl.
3. For two minutes in a large mixing bowl, beat butter with Swerve until light and fluffy. In a separate bowl, whisk together the egg and vanilla extract.
4. Mix in the almond flour until the dough comes together. Form the dough into 3/4-inch balls, then roll them between your palms to form crescents.
5. Bake fifteen to eighteen minutes, or until just faintly golden brown, on prepared baking sheets. They will not be firm when you touch them, but they will harden up as they cool. Allow cooling on the pan.

<u>For the glaze</u>

1. Combine powdered Swerve, 1/4 cup cream, and vanilla extract in a mixing bowl and whisk until smooth. Add 1 tablespoon additional cream at a time until you reach a thin, spreadable consistency.
2. Spread on cooled cookies and top with chosen decorations.
3. Alternatively, simply roll the cookies in powdered sugar.

KETO PEANUT BUTTER BALLS

Prep Time: 20 Minutes

Cook Time: 0 Minutes

Serves: 18-20

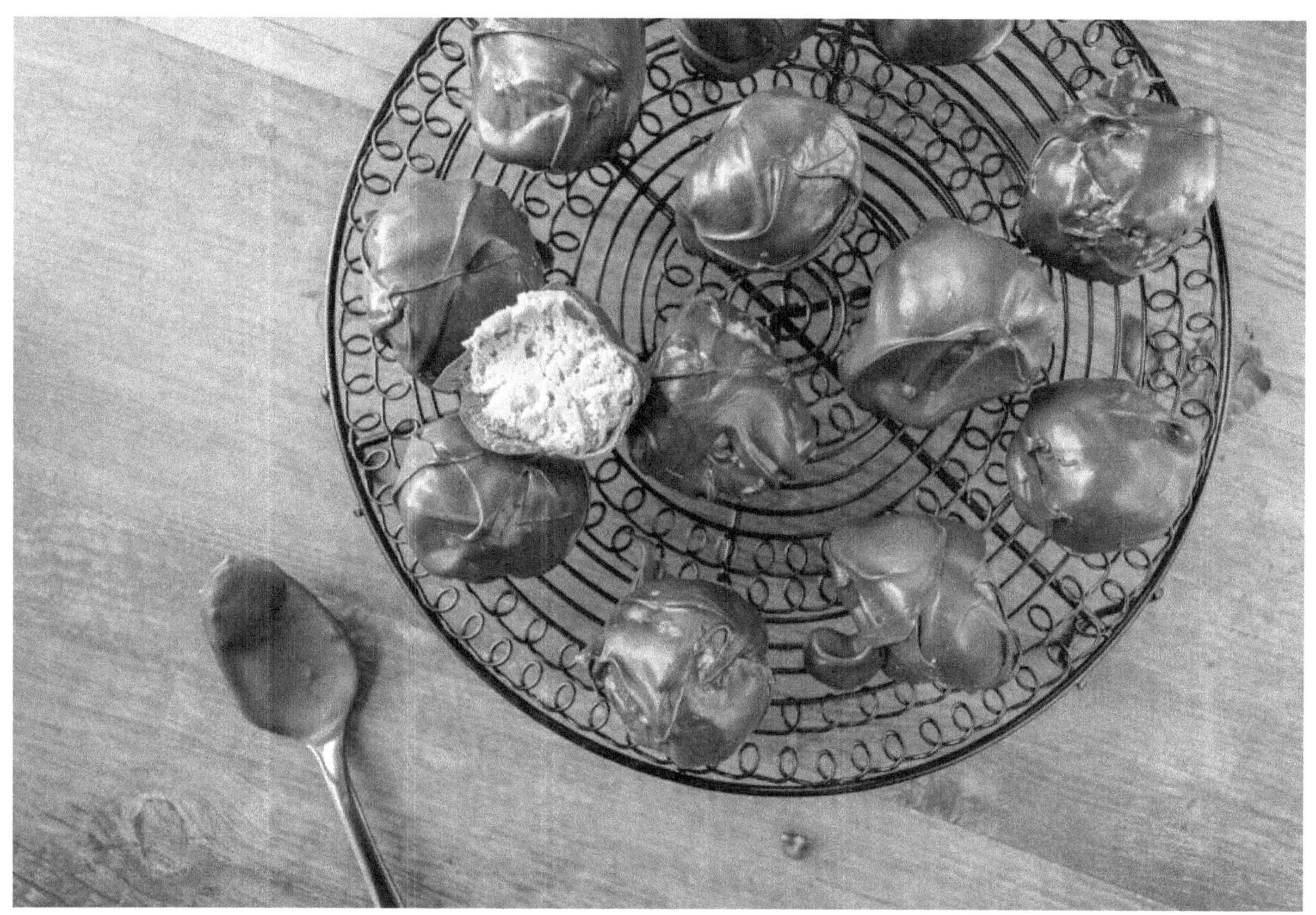

These Keto Peanut Butter Balls are excellent for satisfying your chocolate peanut butter desire with only 4 ingredients

Nutrition

Calories: 194 | Carbohydrates: 7g | Protein: 7g | Fiber: 3g | Sugar: 1g

Fat: 17g | Saturated Fat: 6g | Cholesterol: 0mg

Ingredients

- 1 cup powdered sweetener such as swerve
- 1 cup salted peanuts finely chopped
- 8 oz sugar-free chocolate chips
- 1 cup peanut butter

Instructions

1. Combine the chopped peanuts, peanut butter, and sweetener in a mixing bowl. Form the dough into 18 balls by dividing it into 18 parts. Place on a baking sheet coated with wax paper. Refrigerate until completely chilled.
2. In a microwave or over a double boiler, melt the chocolate chips. Stir chocolate chips every 30 seconds in the microwave until they are 75 percent melted. Then simply mix until all of the remaining ingredients have melted.
3. Place each peanut butter ball back on the wax paper after dipping it in the chocolate. Refrigerate the chocolate until it hardens.

WALNUT SNOWBALL COOKIES

Prep Time: 15 Minutes

Cook Time: 30 Minutes

Serves: 15

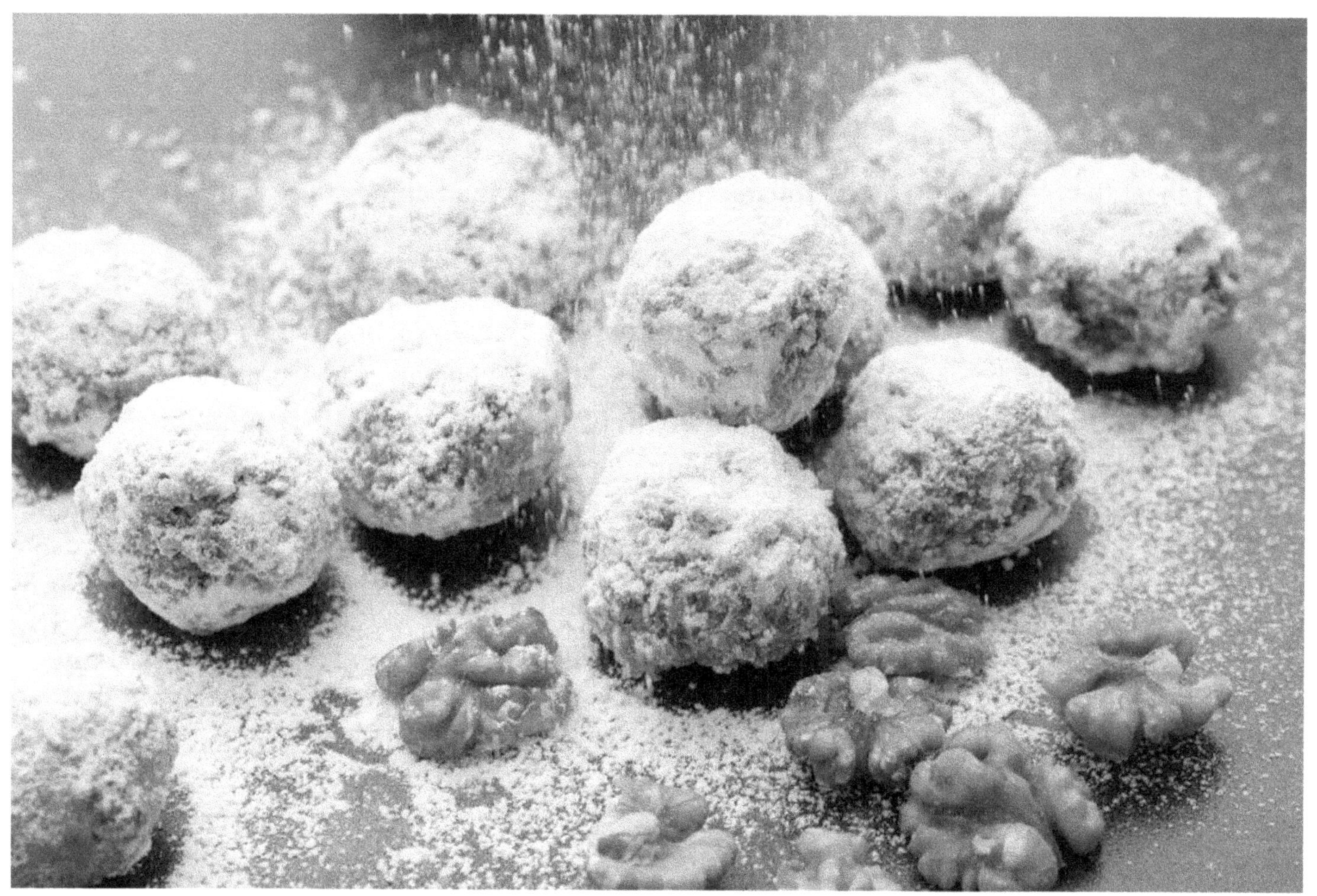

Soft walnut snowball cookies that melt in your tongue. This recipe makes the best Christmas cookies for the holidays

Nutrition

Calories: 127 | Fat: 12g | Saturated Fat: 5g | Fiber: 2g | Sugar: 1g | Protein: 2g

Cholesterol: 29mg | Carbohydrates: 3g

Ingredients

- 1 large Egg
- 1/2 cup swerve confectioner
- 50 drops Liquid Stevia
- 1/2 cup butter, melted
- 1/2 cup Coconut flour
- 1/2 teaspoon vanilla extract
- 1 cup walnuts

Instructions

1. Preheat the oven to 300 degrees Fahrenheit and prepare a baking sheet with parchment paper.
2. In a large bowl, whisk together the melted butter, egg, stevia, and vanilla essence.
3. Pulse the walnuts in a food processor until they are finely ground. In a medium mixing bowl, combine the walnut flour, coconut flour, and 1/4 cup swerve. Combine
4. Add the dry ingredients to the wet mixture in two parts and whisk to incorporate.
5. The dough should be sticky but stiff enough to roll into balls without sticking to your palms at this point. If the consistency isn't appropriate, add 1-2 tablespoons more coconut flour and mix well.
6. Line the parchment paper with 15 equal-sized balls. In the oven, they will not spread. Preheat oven to 350°F and bake for thirty minutes.
7. Allow five minutes for cooling before rolling the balls in the remaining 1/4 cup swerve. Place them back on the parchment paper and set aside for another twenty to thirty minutes to cool completely before eating.

KETO CHOCOLATE MUG CAKE

Prep Time: 5 Minutes

Cook Time: 2 Minutes

Serves: 1

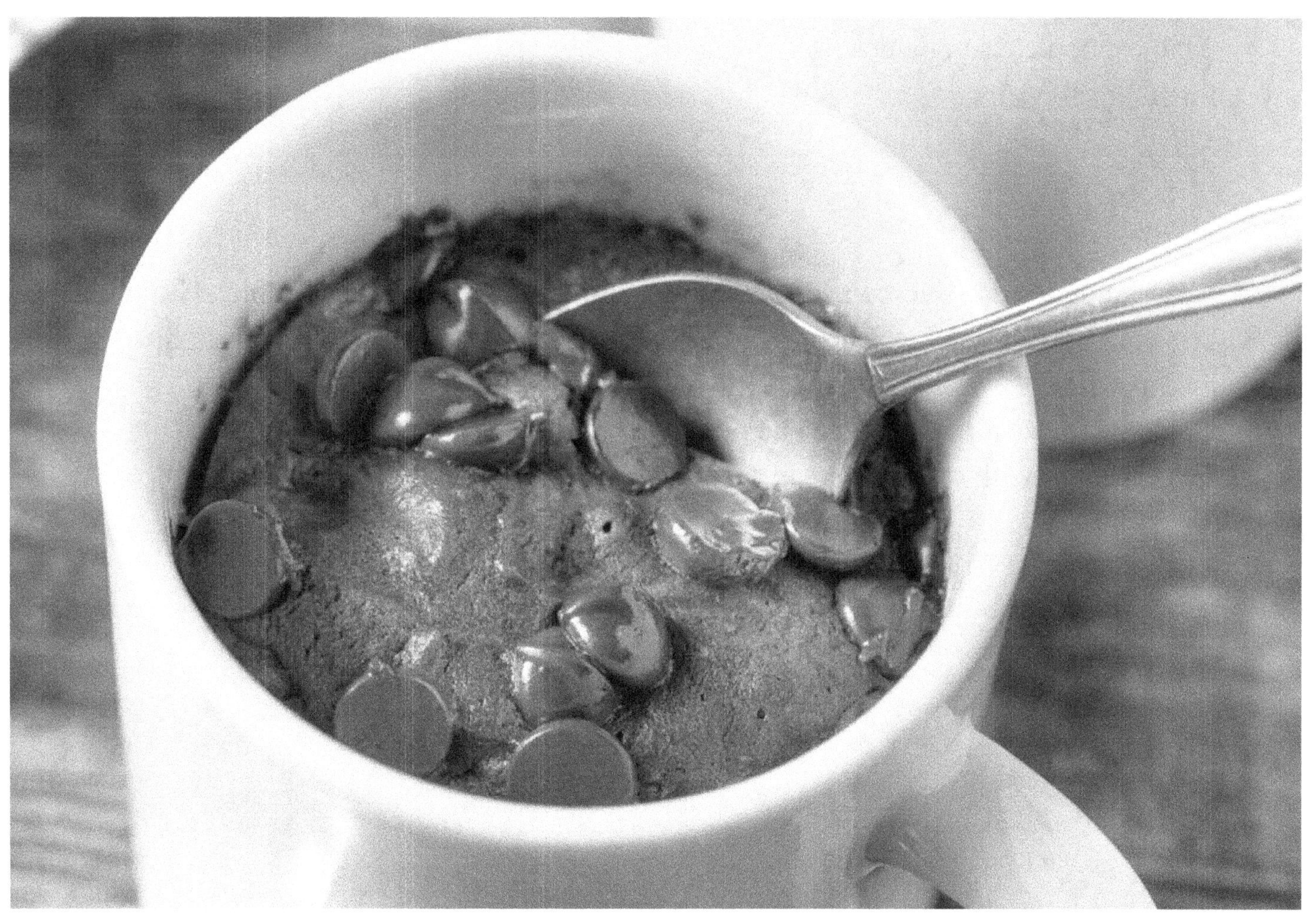

When you have a chocolate craving, you need to act quickly. For such occasions, this chocolate mug cake is ideal. It's made even better by the fact that it's keto. The whole thing is made in a mug, so there's no need to share! It will be ready before your oven has had a chance to preheat.

Nutrition

Calories: 470 | Protein: 15g | Carbohydrates: 8g | Saturated Fat: 18g | Fiber: 7g

Sugar: 1g | Fat: 44g | Sodium: 530mg

Ingredients

- 2 tablespoon butter
- 1/4 cup almond flour
- 1 large egg, beaten
- 2 tablespoon keto-friendly chocolate chips
- 1/4 cup whipped cream for serving
- 2 tablespoon granulated Swerve
- 1/2 teaspoon baking powder
- 2 tablespoon cocoa powder
- Pinch kosher salt

Instructions

1. Heat the butter in a microwave-safe cup for thirty seconds or until completely melted.
2. Stir in the remaining ingredients, excluding the whipped cream, until thoroughly incorporated.
3. Cook for forty-five seconds to one minute, or until the cake is firm but not dry.
4. To serve, top with whipped cream.

KETO PEANUT BUTTER MOUSSE

Prep Time: 5 Minutes

Cook Time: 2 Minutes

Serves: 8

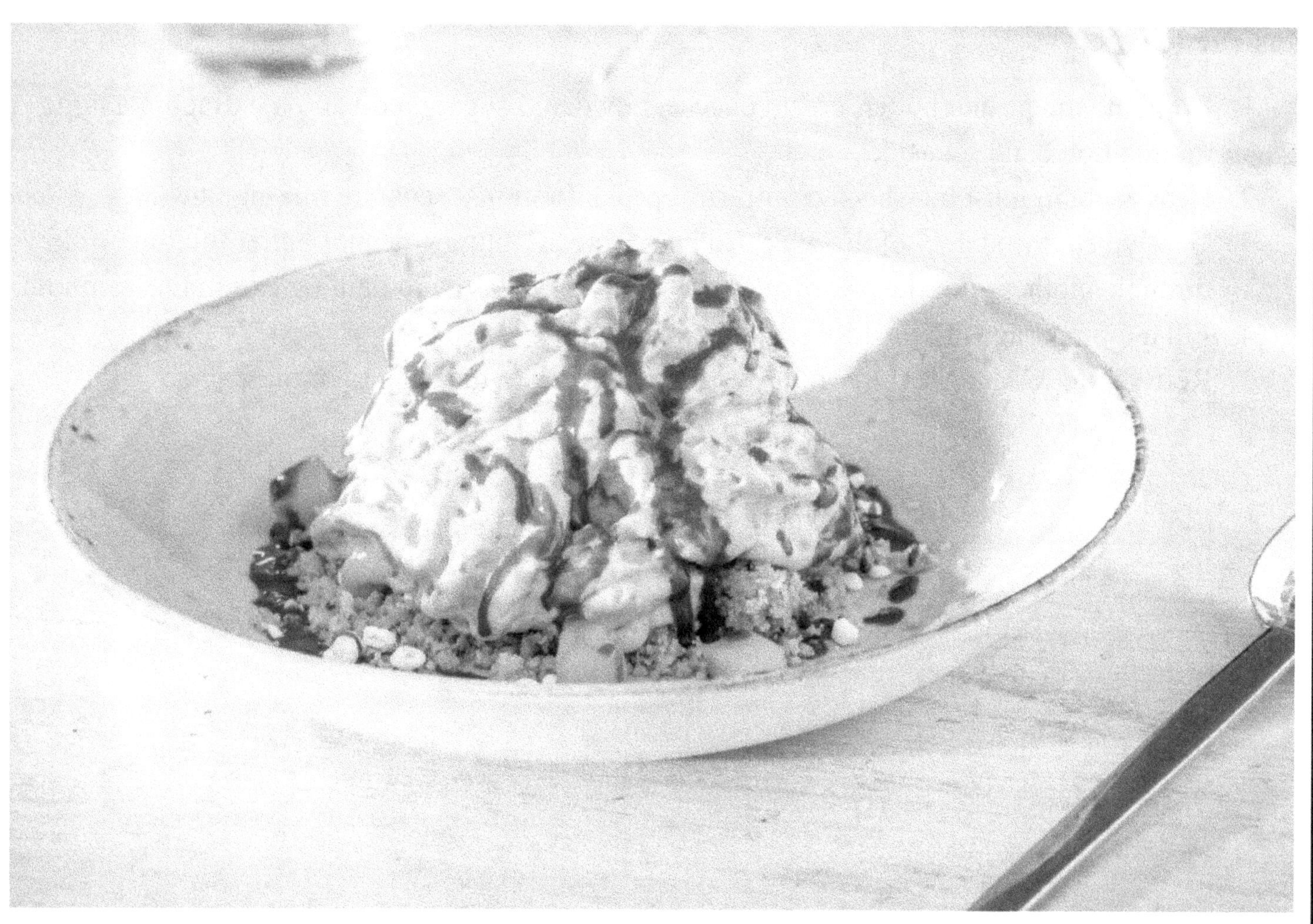

You won't believe this low-carb peanut butter mousse is so light, silky, and creamy! It takes less than 10 minutes to create with only 4 ingredients.

Nutrition

Calories: 288kcal | Carbohydrates: 7g |Net Carbohydrates: 3g | Fiber: 4g |

 Protein: 10g | Fat: 26g | Sodium: 239mg |

Ingredients

- 1 cup heavy cream
- 1 cup peanut butter sugar-free and smooth
- 1 cup sugar-free powdered sugar
- 1 teaspoon vanilla extract optional
- 1 cup cream cheese softened

Instructions

1. Combine the peanut butter, cream cheese, powdered sugar, and vanilla extract in a large mixing bowl and set aside.
2. Heavy cream must be whisked until firm peaks form in a separate mixing bowl.
3. Gently beat through ¼ of the whipped heavy cream into the peanut butter mixture. Fold through another ½ of the cream and mix well. Blend in the remaining cream until smooth.
4. Fill a piping bag with the mousse and a swirly tip.
5. Refrigerate for at least thirty minutes after piping into mason jars or glass jars.

MAGIC KETO COOKIES

Prep Time: 10 Minutes

Cook Time: 15 Minutes

Serves: 15

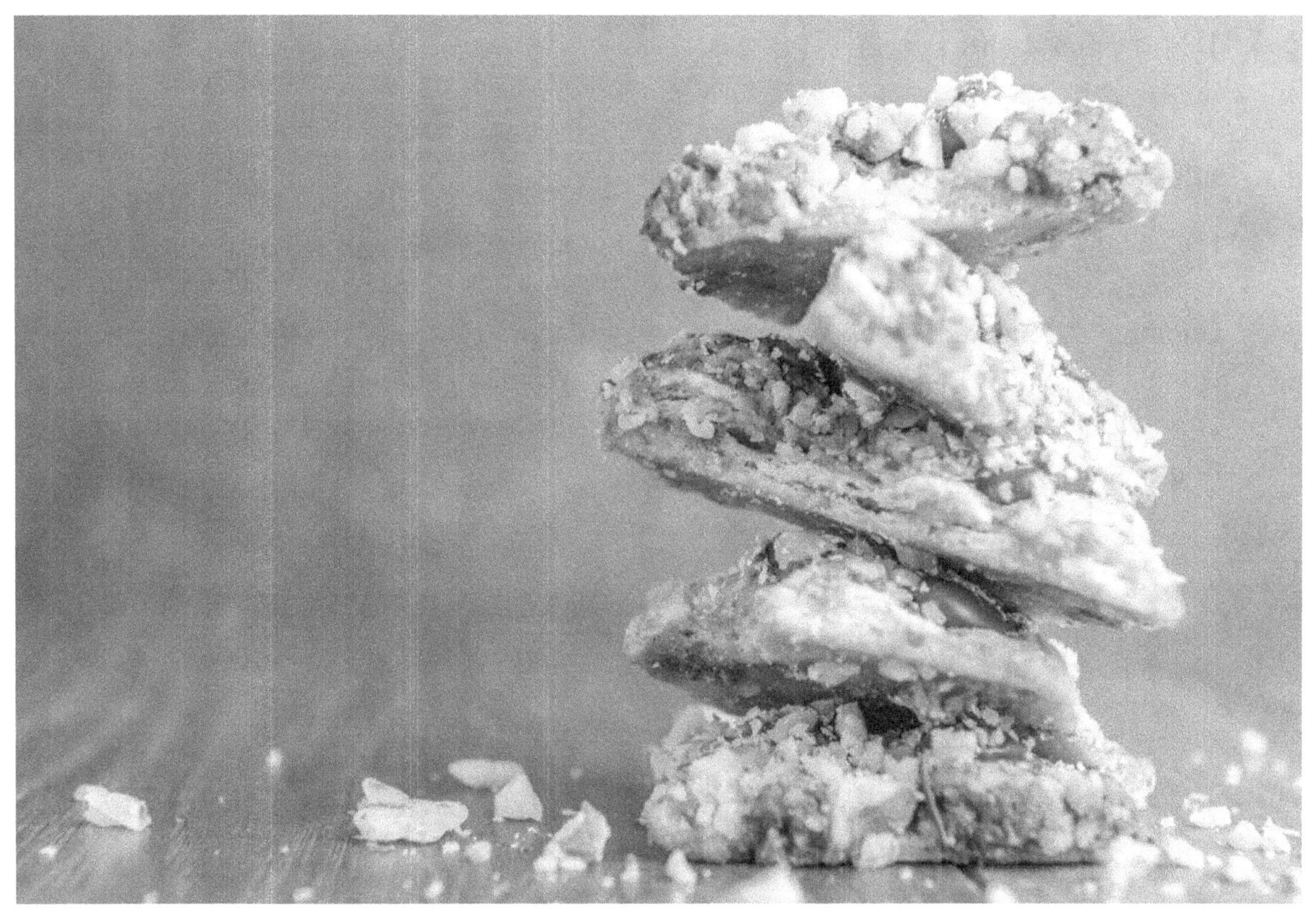

These cookies have a magical quality. Because they're so simple to make and don't contain any flour, you can feel good about having more than one. Make sure your coconut oil and butter aren't melted. Both are at room temperature, but solid, or the cookies will spread when baking.

Nutrition

Calories: 130 | Protein: 2g | Fiber: 1g | Sugar: 0g | Fat: 13g | Carbohydrates: 2g

Saturated Fat: 8g | Sodium: 25mg

Ingredients

- 4 large egg yolks
- 3 tablespoon butter, softened
- 3 tablespoon granulated Swerve sweetener
- 1 cup sugar-free dark chocolate chips
- 3/4 cup roughly chopped walnuts
- 1/4 cup coconut oil
- 1 cup coconut flakes
- 1/2 teaspoon kosher salt

Instructions

1. Preheat the oven to 350 degrees Fahrenheit and prepare a baking sheet with parchment paper.
2. Combine coconut oil, butter, sweetener, salt, and egg yolks in a large mixing dish. Combine chocolate chips, coconut, and walnuts in a mixing bowl.
3. Drop the batter by the tablespoon onto the prepared baking sheet and bake for fifteen minutes, or until golden.

KETO DONUTS WITH A RICH CHOCOLATE GLAZE

Prep Time: 15 Minutes

Cook Time: 15 Minutes

Serves: 10

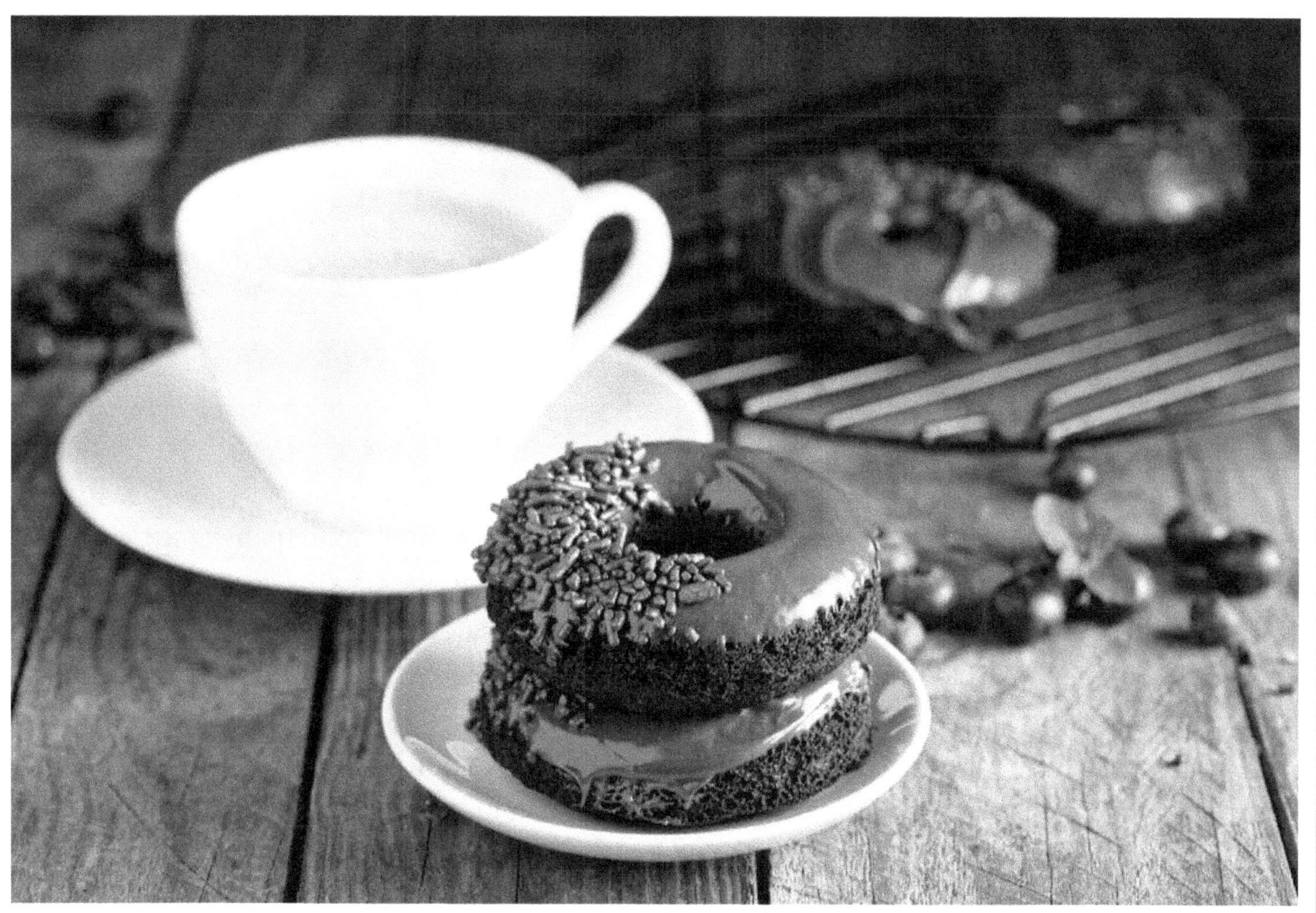

These incredible keto donuts are almost as good as actual cake donuts! They're chocolaty, soft, and moist.

Nutrition

Calories: 221kcal | Carbohydrates: 6g | Fiber: 3g | Sugar: 5g | Protein: 5g

Fat: 17g | Saturated Fat: 11g | Sodium: 116mg

Ingredients

<u>Donuts</u>

- 4 large eggs
- 3 tablespoons whole milk
- ¼ cup unsweetened natural cocoa powder
- ½ cup unsalted butter melted
- Nonstick oil for pan
- 1 teaspoon stevia glycerite
- ¼ teaspoon baking soda
- ¼ cup coconut flour
- ¼ teaspoon sea salt

<u>Glaze</u>

- 1 tablespoon avocado oil
- ¾ cup dark chocolate chips

Instructions

1. Preheat the oven to 350 degrees Fahrenheit. Grease 10 silicone donut pan cavities.
2. Combine the eggs, melted butter, milk, and stevia in a mixing bowl.
3. Mix the coconut flour, cocoa powder, salt, and baking soda in a mixing bowl.
4. Fill the donut pan cavities ¾ full. Bake for seventeen minutes, or until donuts are set and a toothpick inserted in the center comes out clean.
5. Allow for 15 minutes to cool after placing the pan on a cooling rack.
6. Meanwhile, melt the chocolate chips in a small basin in the microwave in 30-second intervals, stirring after each session. Add the avocado oil and mix well.
7. Gently run a knife along the donut's edges and center. Remove the donuts from the pan with care. Dip each donut into the glaze.

THE BEST LOW CARB KETO ICE CREAM

Prep Time: 5 Minutes

Cook Time: 30 Minutes

Chill Time: 4 Hours

Serves: 8

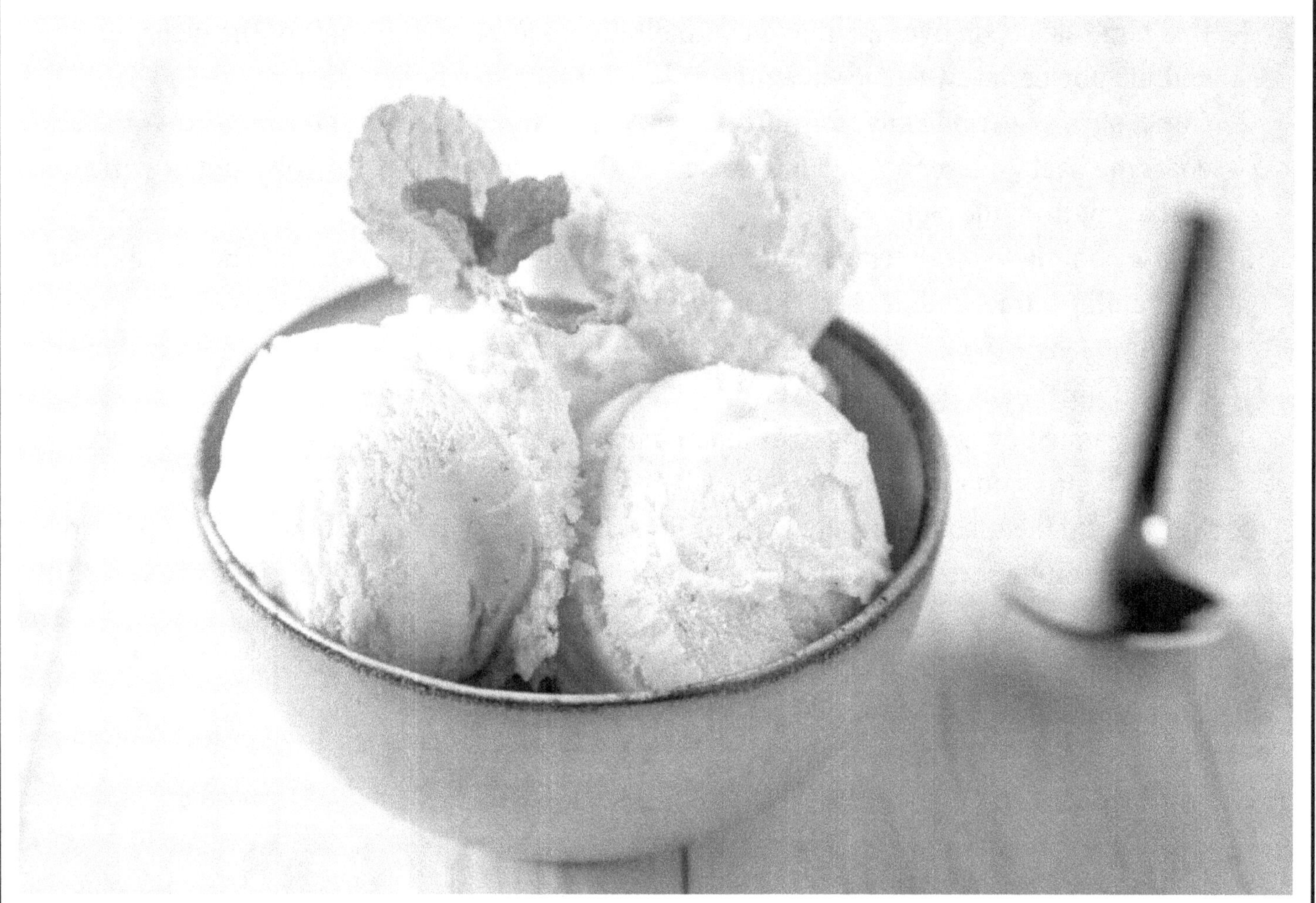

Keto ice cream made with only 4 ingredients! It's the best sugar-free, low-carb ice cream ever.

Nutrition

Calories: 347 | Fat: 36g | Protein: 2g | Fiber: 0g | Sugar: 2g | Total Carbohydrates: 3g

Net Carbohydrates: 3g

Ingredients

- 1/3 cup Besti Powdered Allulose
- 1/4 cup MCT Oil 1 medium Vanilla bean
- 4 cups Heavy cream
- 1 teaspoon Vanilla extract
- 3 tablespoon Butter

Instructions

1. In a large saucepan over medium heat, melt the butter. Combine half of the heavy cream and the powdered sweetener in a mixing bowl. Bring to a boil, then lower to low heat.
2. Cook, stirring periodically, for thirty to forty-five minutes, or until the mixture is thick, coats the back of a spoon, and has decreased in volume by half. As you tilt it, it will also pull away from the pan.
3. Allow cooling to room temperature in a large mixing basin. In a separate bowl, combine the vanilla extract and, if used, the seeds from the vanilla bean. If you don't have an ice cream machine, whisk in the MCT oil or MCT oil powder. This is optional if you have one but highly suggested for texture if you don't.
4. In a separate bowl, whisk together the remaining 2 cups of heavy cream and the sweet mixture until smooth.
5. Refrigerate the mixture for at least four hours or overnight for optimal results. Of course, if you absolutely want to, you can skip this step, but the texture will be better if you chill it.

KETO BLUEBERRY LEMON CHEESECAKE BARS

Prep Time: 30 Minutes

Cook Time: 20 Minutes

Serves: 12

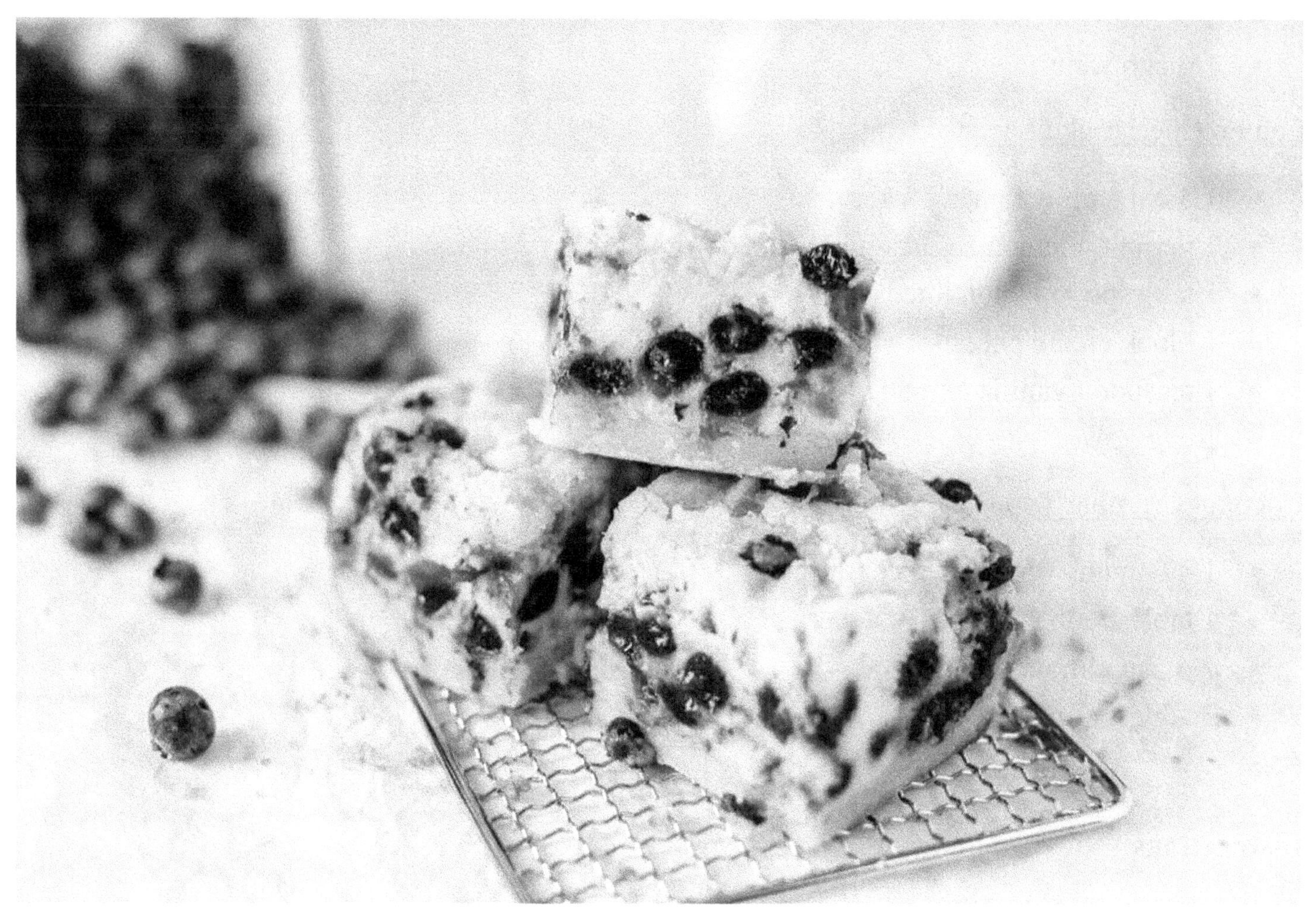

The ultimate four-layer keto dessert is Keto Blueberry Lemon Cheesecake bars! You won't believe how decadent they are at only 5.5 net carbohydrates per bar

Nutrition

Calories: 256 | Total Fat: 19.9g | Cholesterol: 60mg | Fiber: 1.1g | Sugar: 3.2g

Protein: 4g | Sodium: 67.2mg

Ingredients

Almond Flour Crust

- 1/3 cup of confectioners swerve sweetener
- 2 tablespoons swerve sweetener
- 1 1/4 cup almond flour
- Low Carb Blueberry Sauce
- 8 tablespoons butter
- 1 1/2 cup blueberries
- 1/4 cup water

Lemon Cheesecake Layer

- 1/3 cup confectioner's swerve
- 1 teaspoon lemon zest, tightly packed
- 1 tablespoon lemon juice
- 1 block cream cheese
- 1 teaspoon vanilla extract
- 1 egg yolk

Coconut Crumble Topping

- 1/4 cup unsweetened coconut flakes
- 1 tablespoon swerve sweetener
- 1/4 cup almond flour
- 2 tablespoons butter

Instructions

To begin preparing the Blueberry Sauce

Combine blueberries, swerve sweeteners, and water in a blender. Allow the mixture to simmer for ten-fifteen minutes or until it thickens. Set aside.

For the Crust

1. Preheat the oven to 350 degrees Fahrenheit.
2. Use foil or parchment paper to line an 8x8 pan.
3. In a small bowl, combine the melted butter, almond flour, and swerve, and press into the foil-lined pan.
4. Prebake the crust for seven minutes or until it begins to color around the edges but is not solid.

5. Remove the crust and set it aside to cool. While the cheesecake layer is still hot, do not add it.

For the Lemon Cheesecake Layer

1. Combine the cream cheese, egg yolk, sweetener, lemon juice, zest, and extract in an electric mixer or small blender until smooth.
2. Evenly spread the cheesecake layer on top of the crust.

For the Blueberry Layer

Over the cheesecake mixture, spread the low-carb blueberry sauce that has been prepared.

For the Crumble

1. In a small blender or food processor, combine the butter, almond flour, unsweetened coconut, and sweetener and pulse until a crumb-like consistency form.
2. Sprinkle blueberries on top of the blueberry layer.
3. Bake for eighteen-twenty minutes, or until lightly browned on top.
4. Allow for complete cooling before slicing.

KETO CHEESECAKE BROWNIES

Prep Time: 10 Minutes

Cook Time: 45 Minutes

Serves: 18

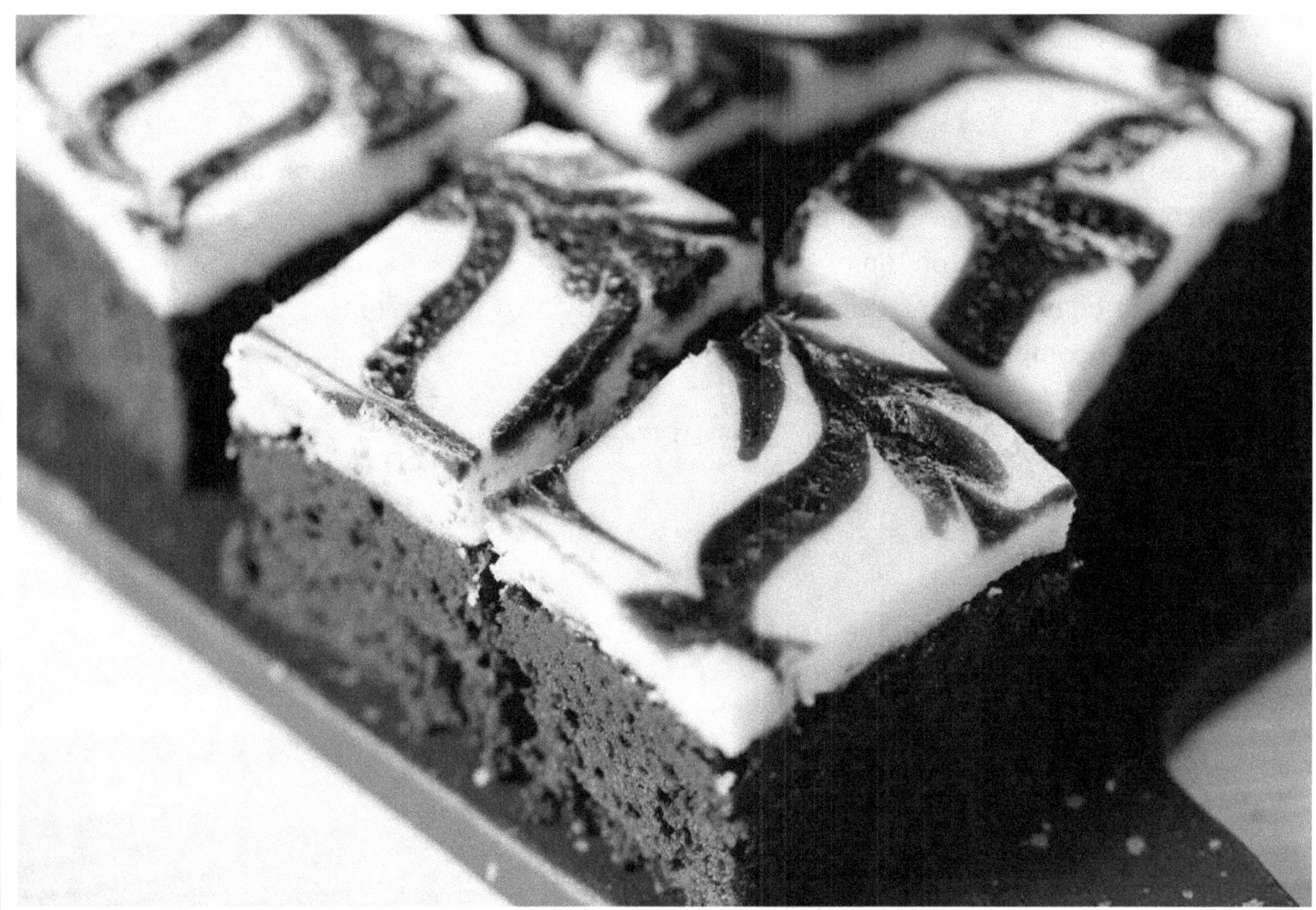

The best keto dessert is these keto cheesecake brownies! A flourless brownie is a bottom layer, which is topped with a sugar-free cheesecake.

Nutrition

Calories: 138 | Sugar: 1g | Fat: 13g | Fiber: 2g | Protein: 4g

Carbohydrates: 4g

Ingredients

<u>Brownie Layer</u>

- 4 eggs, at room temperature
- 4 teaspoons vanilla extract
- 6 tablespoons melted butter or coconut oil
- 1 cup swerve sweetener or coconut sugar
- 1 cup unsweetened cocoa powder
- Pinch of sea salt

<u>Cheesecake Layer</u>

- 1/3 cup plus 2 tablespoons swerve sweetener or coconut sugar
- 8 ounces organic cream cheese, at room temperature
- 2 organic eggs, at room temperature
- 1/2 tablespoon vanilla extract
- 1/3 cup sour cream
- 1/3 cup heavy cream

Instructions

<u>Brownie Layer</u>

1. Preheat oven to 350 degrees Fahrenheit.
2. Mix the dry ingredients in a mixing bowl.
3. Add the eggs one at a time, mixing well after each addition.
4. Combine the melted coconut oil and vanilla extract in a bowl and mix.
5. Mix thoroughly and pour into a buttered 8-inch baking pan.
6. Bake the brownies for fifteen-twenty minutes, or until a toothpick inserted in the center comes out clean.

<u>Cheesecake Layer</u>

1. Combine all of the ingredients in a mixing bowl and whisk until smooth.
2. The cream cheese must be at room temperature to avoid chunking. If your cream cheese isn't soft enough, use a stick blender to smooth out the mixture.
3. Over the baked and slightly cooled brownie layer, pour the cheesecake mix.
4. Bake for another twenty-five to thirty minutes, or until the cheesecake layer is lightly browned.
5. Allow for many hours of cooling before serving.
6. Serve by cutting into squares.

KETO SOPAPILLA CHEESECAKE BARS

Prep Time: 15 Minutes

Cook Time: 50 Minutes

Serves: 16

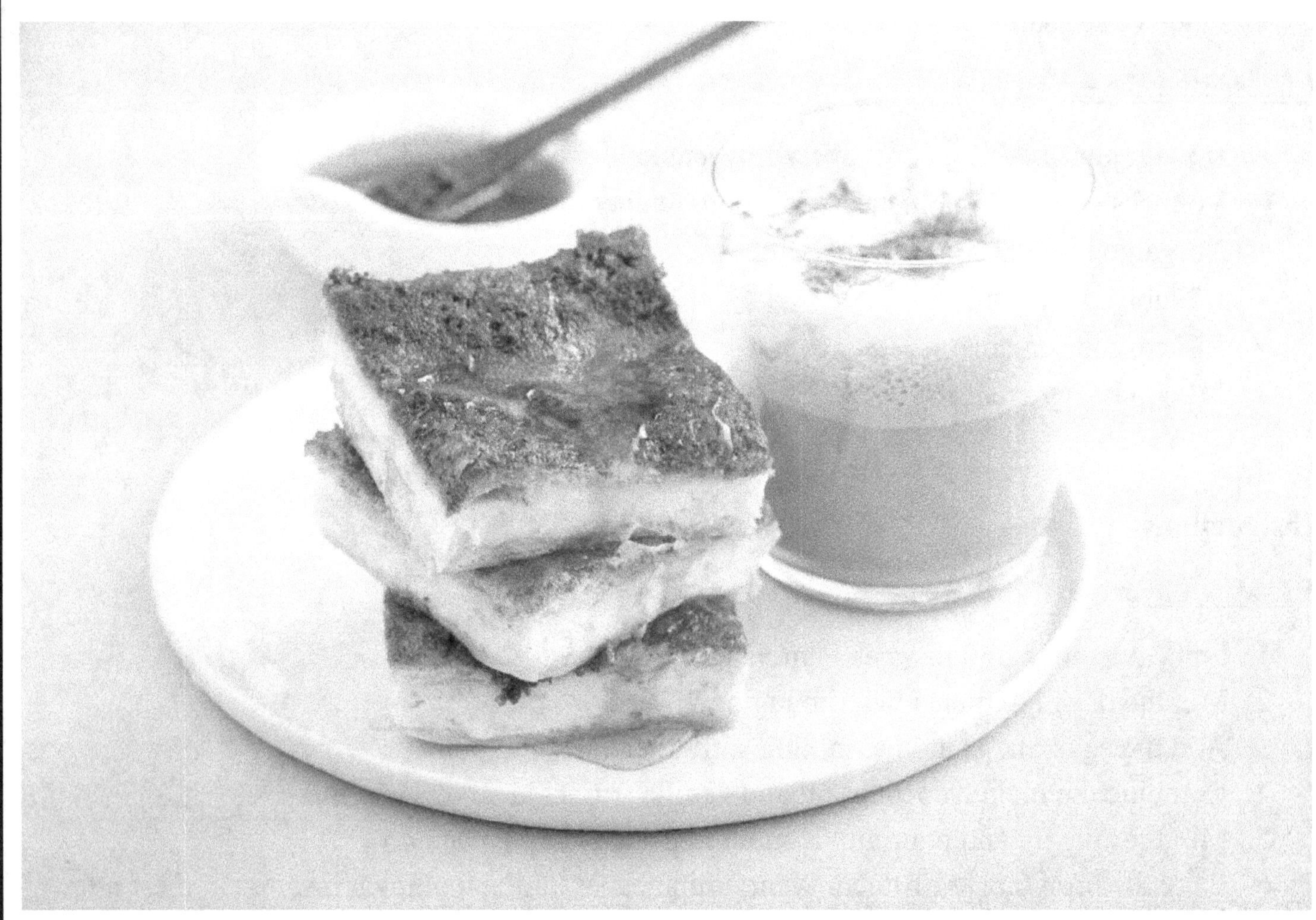

Bars of Sopapilla Cheesecake are surrounded by layers of soft, slightly sweet dough that are sprinkled with cinnamon. Because no plates or forks are required, these are ideal for sharing.

Nutrition

Calories: 190 | Carbohydrates: 4g | Fiber: 1g | Sugar: 1g | Protein: 6g

Fat: 16g | Saturated Fat: 8g | Cholesterol: 76mg

Ingredients

<u>Dough</u>

- 1 egg
- 2 tablespoon Joy Filled Eats Sweetener
- 8 oz mozzarella shredded or cubed
- ⅓ cup almond flour
- ⅓ cup coconut flour
- 2 oz cream cheese
- 1 teaspoon baking powder
- 1 teaspoon vanilla

<u>Cheesecake Filling</u>

- 2 eggs
- ½ cup Joy Filled Eats Sweetener
- 14 oz cream cheese
- 1 teaspoon vanilla

<u>Cinnamon Topping</u>

- 2 tablespoon Joy Filled Eats Sweetener
- 2 tablespoon melted butter
- 1 tablespoon cinnamon

Instructions

1. Preheat the oven to 350 degrees Fahrenheit.
2. In a microwave-safe bowl, place the cheese. 1 minute in the microwave Stir.
3. Microwave thirty seconds Stir. All of the cheese should be melted at this stage. Microwave for another thirty seconds, or until the mixture is homogeneous and gloopy; it should resemble cheese fondue at this stage.
4. In a food processor, combine the other dough ingredients as well as the cheese. Using the dough blade, blend until a consistent hue is achieved. Wet your hands and press half of it into an 8x8 baking dish once it has reached a uniform color. On a piece of parchment paper, press out the other half into an 8x8 square.
5. To create the cheesecake filling, combine the cream cheese, vanilla, eggs, and sweetener in a food processor no need to clean or a mixing bowl. Then, in a food processor or with an electric mixer, blend until smooth.

6. On top of the bottom layer of dough, pour the cheesecake batter. Remove the parchment paper and gently place the other square of dough on top. Drizzle the melted butter over the top and sprinkle the sugar and cinnamon on top.
7. Preheat oven to 350°F and bake for fifty-sixty minutes, or until golden brown and puffy. If the butter pools in the center, use a pastry brush to brush it over the top during the final twenty minutes of baking.
8. Cover the top with foil if it starts to brown too much.

KETO AVOCADO POPS

Prep Time: 5 Minutes

Cook Time: 5 Minutes

Serves: 10

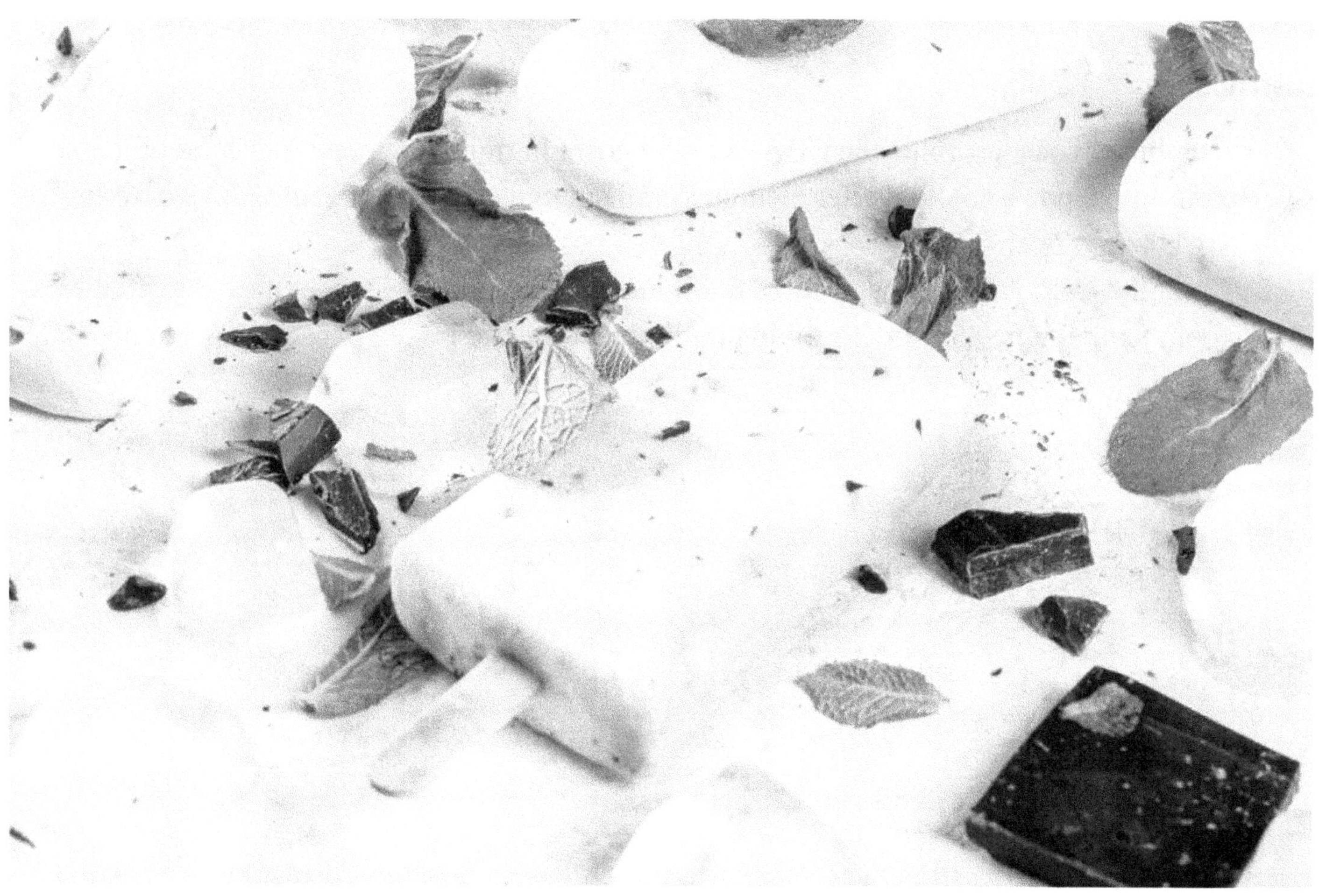

If you're not on a keto diet but still want to try these pops, replace the real sugar with maple syrup or agave nectar

Nutrition

Calories: 120 | Protein: 1g | Fiber: 3g | Sugar: 0g | Fat: 12g | Carbohydrates: 5g

Saturated Fat: 5g | Sodium: 5mg

Ingredients

- 3 tablespoon Swerve or other sugar alternatives
- 3/4 cup coconut milk
- 1 cup keto-friendly chocolate
- 3 ripe avocados
- 1 tablespoon coconut oil
- Juice of 2 limes

Instructions

1. Combine avocados, lime juice, Swerve, and coconut milk in a blender or food processor. Pour into a popsicle mold after blending until smooth. Freeze until firm, anywhere from six hours to overnight.
2. Combine chocolate chips and coconut oil in a medium mixing dish. Allow it to cool to room temperature after microwaving until melted. Serve frozen pops dipped in chocolate.

KETO CHOCOLATE TRUFFLES

Prep Time: 10 Minutes

Cook Time: 2 Minutes

Chill Time: 20 Minutes

Serves: 15

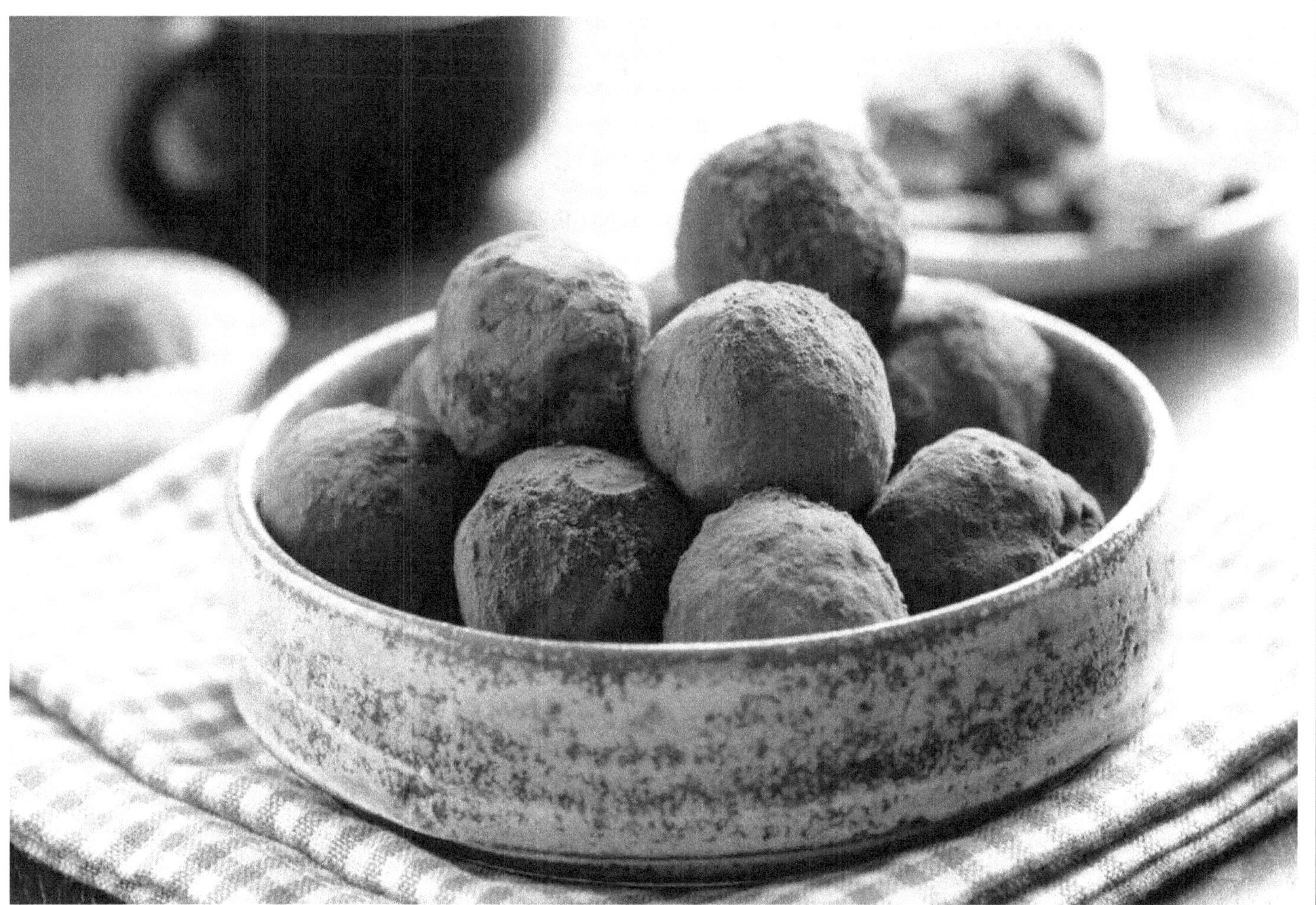

These keto chocolate truffles are velvety smooth, decadently rich, and really easy to create — the ideal low-carb chocolate dessert.

Nutrition

Calories: 20kcal | Protein: 1g | Fiber: 1g | Sugar: 0g | Fat: 2g | Carbohydrates: 2g

Saturated Fat: 0g | Sodium: 35mg

Ingredients

- 1 medium avocado, mashed
- 1 cup dark chocolate chips, melted
- 1 teaspoon vanilla extract
- 1/4 cup cocoa powder
- 1/4 teaspoon Kosher salt

Instructions

1. Combine melted chocolate, avocado, vanilla, and salt in a medium mixing bowl. Stir everything together until it's smooth and well blended. Place in the refrigerator for fifteen to twenty minutes to firm up somewhat.
2. Use a small cookie scoop or a small spoon to scoop roughly 1 tablespoon chocolate mixture once it has set. Roll the chocolate in your palm until it is circular, then roll it in cocoa powder.

KETO BLUEBERRY CHOCOLATE CLUSTERS

Prep Time: 5 Minutes

Cook Time: 5 Minutes

Chill Time: 15 Minutes

Serves: 12

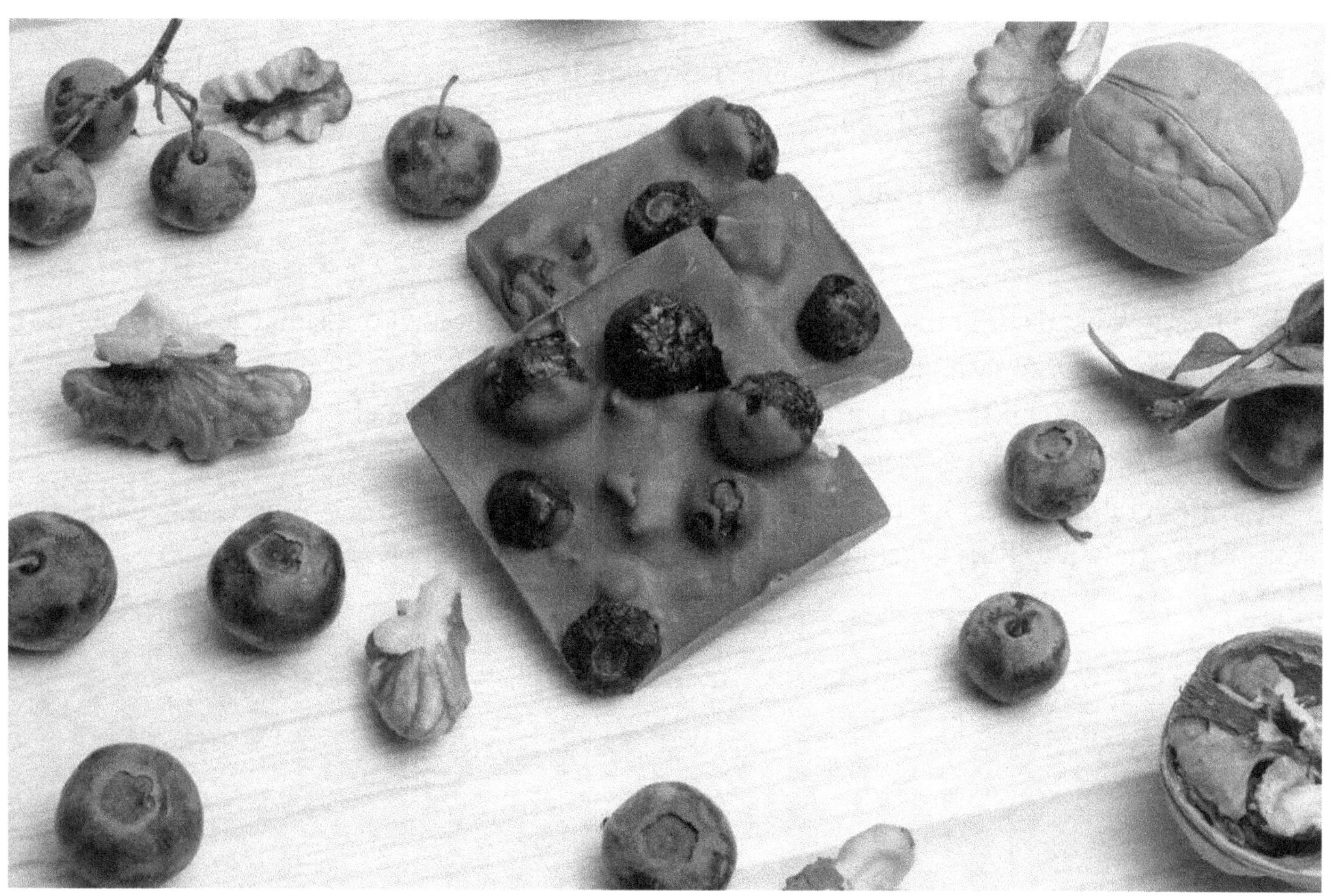

Chocolate cravings may be satisfied in minutes with these raspberry and blueberry chocolate clusters! They're the ultimate low-carb snack since they're packed with healthy fats and low-sugar fruit that you'll want to eat right away.

Nutrition

Calories: 61kcal | Fat: 6g | Saturated Fat: 4.7g | Fiber: 1.3g | Sugar: 0.7g | Protein: 0.4g

Cholesterol: 0mg | Salt: 50mg | Carbohydrates: 3.2g | Net Carbohydrates: 1.9g

Ingredients

- 1 tablespoon non-GMO erythritol, birch xylitol
- 1-1.5 cups fresh blueberries or raspberries
- 4 tablespoons coconut butter
- 2 tablespoons cacao powder
- 2 tablespoons cacao butter
- 1 tablespoon coconut oil
- Pinch of salt

<u>Optional</u>

- Raw chopped nuts or chopped Collagen Protein Bars
- Shredded unsweetened coconut

Instructions

1. Over low heat, stir in the coconut butter, cacao butter, coconut oil, salt, cacao powder, and sweetener to taste until completely melted.
2. Fill a silicone muffin pan with at least 12 parts evenly with the chocolate mixture. Sprinkle berries and any other mix-ins, if used, evenly over the chocolate.
3. Refrigerate the trays for fifteen minutes to allow them to set.
4. Enjoy right away. Refrigerate leftovers in an airtight container.

CARROT CAKE BITES

Prep Time: 5 Minutes

Cook Time: 15 Minutes

Serves: 10

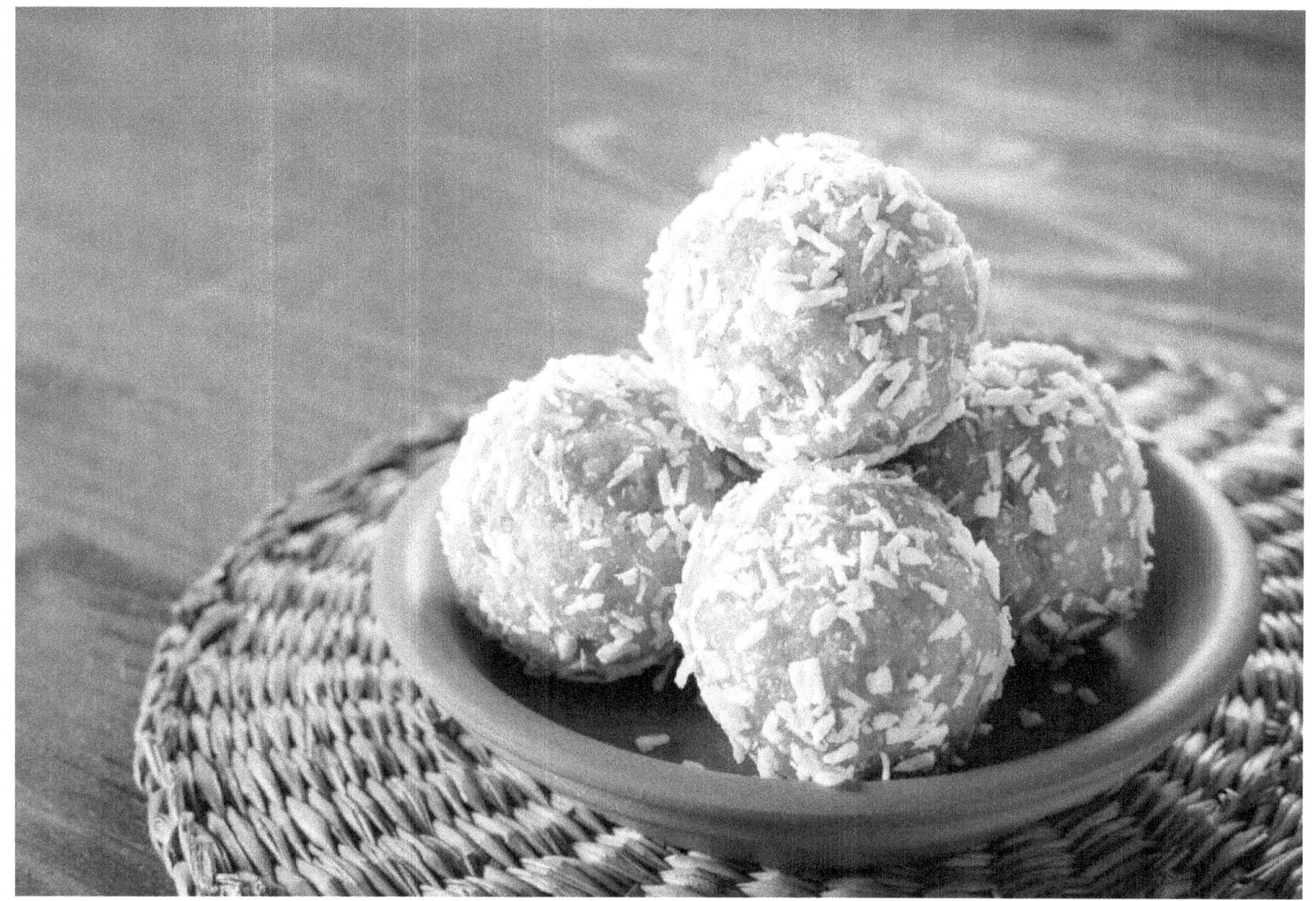

Spring has here in full force! These carrot cake bites are the ideal springtime snack! It's perfect for Easter or any other springtime gathering. Paleo, low-carb, keto, dairy-free, and sugar-free diets are all options.

Nutrition

Calories: 50 | Fat: 4g | Fiber: 1g | Sugar: 1g | Net Carbohydrates: 1g

Total Carbohydrates: 3g | Protein: 1g

Ingredients

- 1 egg
- 1 tablespoon sweetener of choice
- 1/2 large carrot, shredded or chopped finely
- 2 tablespoons butter or coconut oil, melted
- 2 tablespoons shredded coconut, no sugar added
- 1/4 cup coconut flour
- 1/8 teaspoon ground nutmeg

Instructions

1. Preheat the oven to 350 degrees Fahrenheit.
2. In a mixing dish, combine all ingredients except the shredded coconut. If the dough is too sticky, add a little more coconut flour. If the mixture is too dry, drizzle in a little extra coconut oil or butter.
3. Divide the mixture into ten equal parts and roll into balls. If desired, roll the balls in shredded coconut.
4. Bake for fifteen to twenty minutes, or until the shredded coconut begins to brown, on a baking sheet.

EASY KETO CHOCOLATE COVERED STRAWBERRIES

Prep Time: 10 Minutes

Cook Time: 1 Minute

Serves: 6

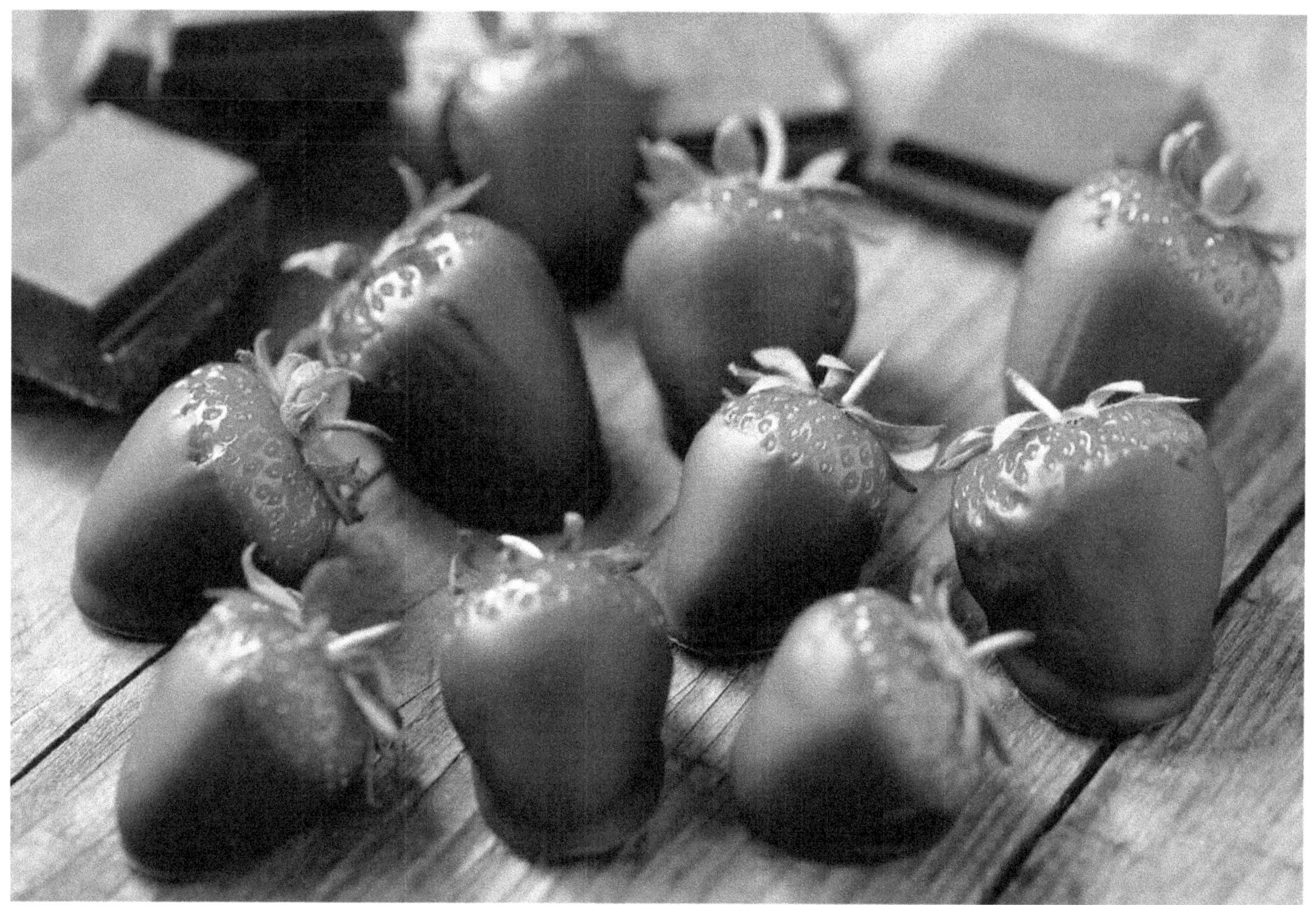

Everything, especially strawberries, tastes better when they've been dipped in chocolate. These sugar-free keto chocolate-covered strawberries can be created in minutes and are the perfect low-carb dessert to share or keep all to yourself.

Nutrition

Calories: 24kcal | Protein: 0.1g | Net Carbohydrates: 1.2g | Fat: 1.8g

Ingredients

- 1 cup keto chocolate chips
- 24 large strawberries
- pink or red food coloring (optional)

Instructions

1. Wash strawberries and let air dry completely or pat dry. If the chocolate is entirely dry, it will attach better to the strawberries.
2. Microwave the chocolate in a small glass bowl for thirty seconds at a time, stirring after each until melted. If you don't want to use the microwave, you can melt your chocolate in a double boiler.
3. Stir in food coloring if using sugar-free white chocolate chips.
4. To dip the strawberries, grasp them by the stems and dip them into molten chocolate. Turn the strawberries so that the chocolate is on all sides. To harden, place on a sheet of parchment or wax paper.

KETO SNICKERDOODLE CRÈME COOKIES

Prep Time: 10 Minutes

Cook Time:12 Minutes

Serves: 18

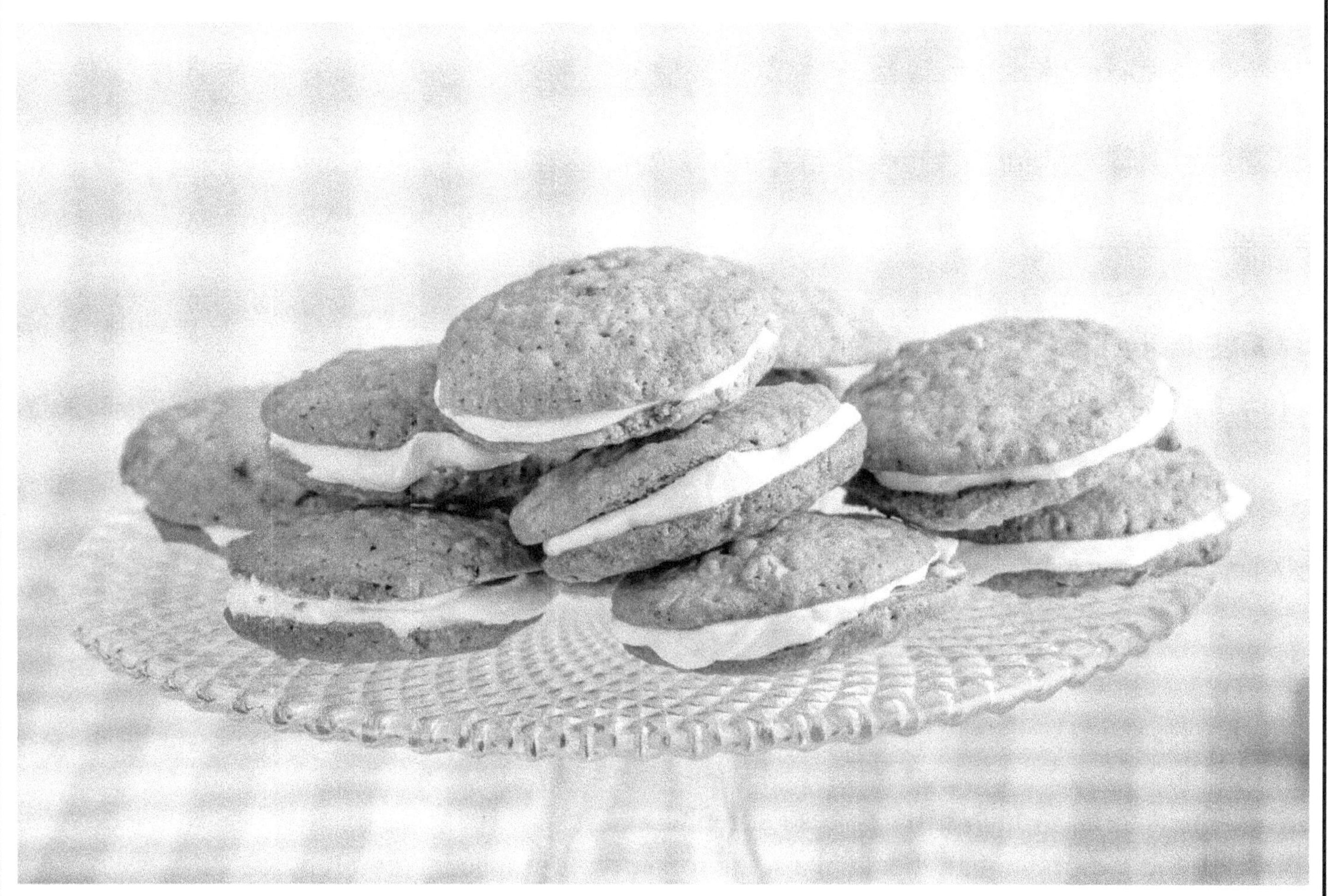

Snickerdoodle Crème Cookies have been given a healthy, sugar-free makeover! You can now enjoy the deliciousness of a conventional cookie without the guilt of Carbohydrates. They're creme-filled and tasty, yet they're so low in Carbohydrates that you can eat a few without worrying about a blood sugar surge.

Nutrition

Calories: 126kcal | Protein: 1.8g | Fiber: 2.7g | Total Fat: 11.4g | Carbohydrate: 4.7g

Cholesterol: 47mg

Ingredients

<u>Cookie</u>

- 2 eggs
- 3/4 teaspoon cream of tartar
- 1 cup coconut flour
- 1/2 cup butter, softened
- 2 teaspoon cinnamon
- 2 teaspoon vanilla extract
- 1 teaspoon baking soda
- 1 cup Swerve
- 1/2 teaspoon salt

<u>Outing Coating</u>

- 1/2 teaspoon cinnamon
- Surkin Gold brown sugar sub

<u>Filling</u>

- 2 tablespoon milk
- 1/2 cup butter, softened
- 1 cup Confectioners Swerve
- 1 teaspoon vanilla extract

Instructions

1. Preheat the oven to 350 degrees Fahrenheit.
2. Blend the first 6 ingredients in a stand mixer on low speed to combine.
3. Blend in the eggs, vanilla, and butter until everything is well combined. Roll into balls with a 1-inch cookie scoop and place on a baking sheet lined with parchment or Silpat.
4. Make 72 balls in total. Roll each one in brown sugar substitute or cinnamon granulated Swerve.
5. Bake for 12 minutes after slightly flattening the balls.
6. Allow it to cool completely.
7. Fill a stand mixer halfway with ingredients and beat on high until smooth.
8. Spread half of the cookies with the filling, then top with another cookie to make 36 sandwich cookies.

LOW CARB CINNAMON ROLL MUG CAKE

Prep Time: 5 Minutes

Cook Time: 1 Minute

Serves: 1

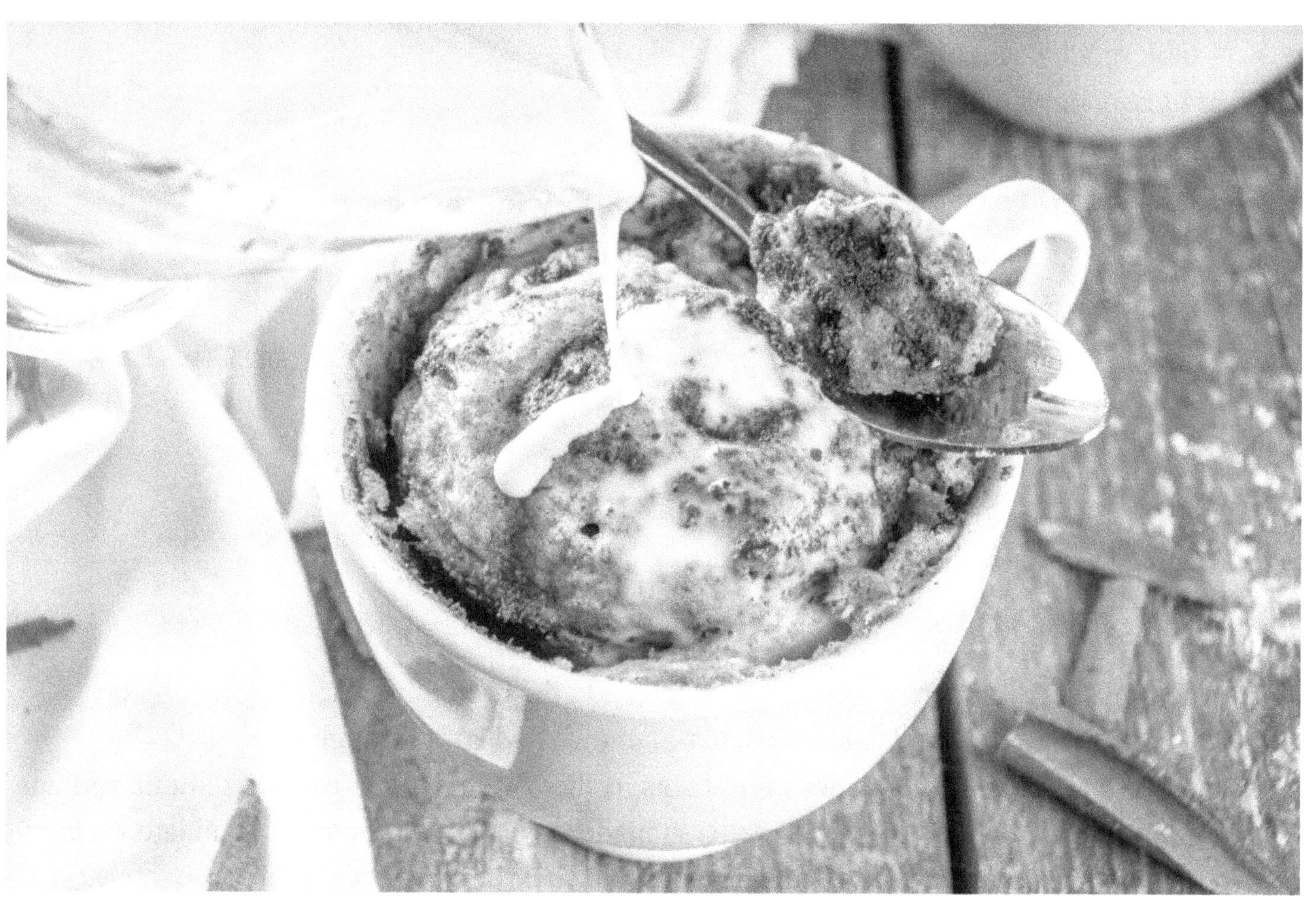

This cinnamon roll-inspired mug cake is extremely fluffy and moist, packed with protein and low in Carbohydrates, and ready in under a minute! This gluten-free, vegan, paleo and sugar-free 1 Minute Low Carb Cinnamon Roll Mug Cake is also naturally gluten-free, vegan, and paleo

Nutrition

Calories: 132kcal | Carbohydrates: 6g | Fat: 4g | Fiber: 253g | Protein: 25g

Ingredients

- 1 large egg
- 1 scoop vanilla protein powder 32-34 grams
- 1/4 cup milk of choice I used unsweetened almond
- 1 tablespoon granulated sweetener of choice
- 1 teaspoon granulated sweetener of choice
- 1/2 teaspoon baking powder
- 1 tablespoon coconut butter melted
- 1 tablespoon coconut flour
- 1/4 teaspoon vanilla extract
- 1/2 teaspoon cinnamon
- 1/2 teaspoon cinnamon(extra)

For the glaze

- pinch cinnamon
- 1/2 teaspoon milk of choice
- 1 tablespoon coconut butter melted

Instructions

For the microwave option

1. Cooking sprays a microwave-safe dish, then add the protein powder, baking powder, coconut flour, cinnamon, and sweetener of choice and stir thoroughly.
2. Mix the egg/whites into the dry ingredients. If the batter is too crumbly, continue adding milk of choice until a fairly thick batter is made. Swirl in your favorite granulated sugar and more cinnamon. Microwave for sixty seconds, or until the center is barely done. Enjoy the glaze on top.

For the oven option

Follow the steps above, but bake for eight-fifteen minutes at 350 degrees Fahrenheit, depending on the consistency desired- A toothpick inserted into the center of the mug cake should come out 'just' clean.

NO-BAKE KETO COCONUT CRACK BARS

Prep Time: 3 Minutes

Cook Time: 3 Minutes

Serves: 20

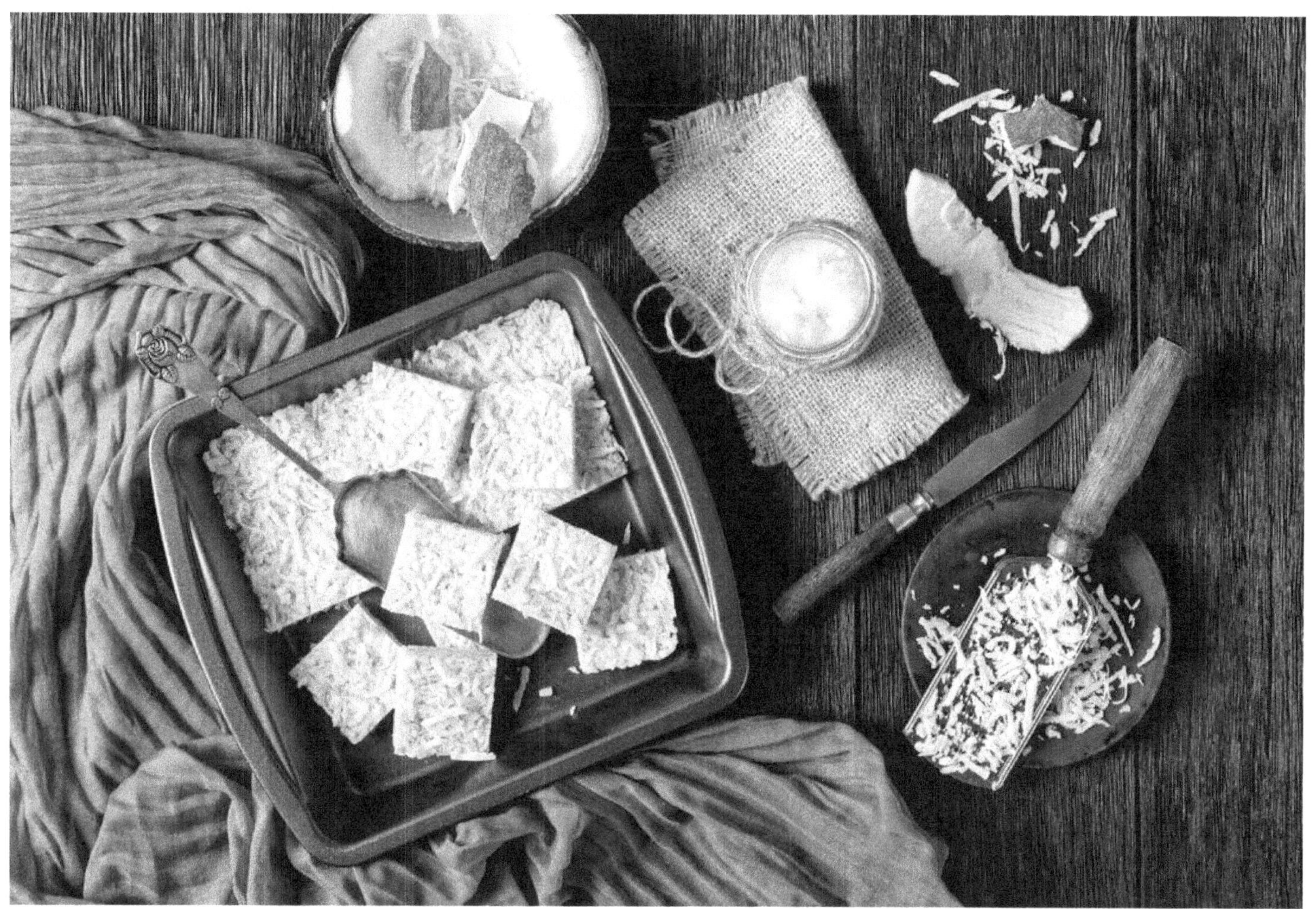

This healthy 3-ingredient dish will satisfy your sweet tooth! These sugar-free, low-carb, keto-friendly coconut bars are really addictive and only take a few minutes to make.

Nutrition

Calories: 108kcal | Carbohydrates: 2g | Fiber: 2g | Iron: 0.2mg | Protein: 2g

Fat: 11g | Sodium: 3mg

Ingredients

- 1/4 cup monk fruit sweetened maple syrup
- 3 cups shredded unsweetened coconut flakes
- 1 cup coconut oil, melted

Instructions

1. Set aside an 8 x 8-inch or 8 x 10-inch pan lined with parchment paper. Alternatively, a loaf pan can be used.
2. Add the shredded unsweetened coconut to a large mixing basin. Mix in the melted coconut oil and monk fruit sweetened maple syrup or your preferred sticky sweetener until a thick batter form. Add a little more syrup or a splash of water if it's too crumbly.
3. Fill the lined pan halfway with the coconut crack bar mixture. Wet your hands lightly and press firmly into place. Freeze or refrigerate until hard. Enjoy by cutting into bars.

KETO VANILLA CUPCAKES

Prep Time: 5 Minutes

Cook Time: 20 Minutes

Serves: 10

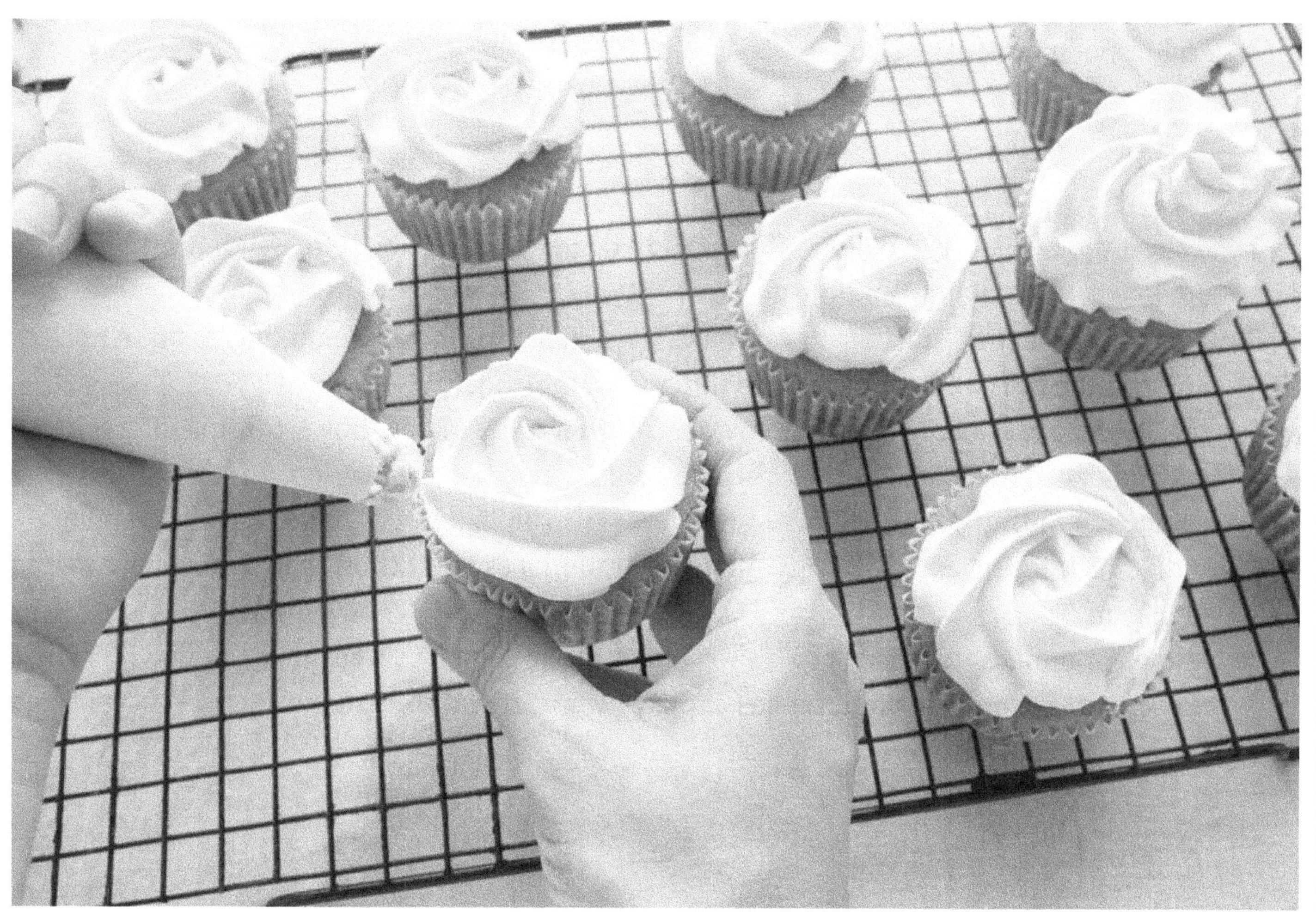

These low-carb, sugar-free cupcakes have a beautiful vanilla taste and are so moist, fluffy, and tender that you won't believe they're low-carb! These keto vanilla cupcakes are easy to make and have keto icing on top.

Nutrition

Calories: 153kcal | Carbohydrates: 4g | Fiber: 2g | Protein: 5g | Fat: 13g | Sodium: 189mg

Potassium: 41mg | Net Carbohydrates: 2g

Ingredients

- 2/3 cup granulated sweetener of choice
- 6 large eggs whisked
- 1/2 cup coconut flour
- 1 teaspoon baking powder
- 1/2 cup butter
- 1 batch keto vanilla frosting
- 2 teaspoon vanilla extract
- 2 tablespoon milk of choice

Instructions

1. Preheat the oven to 180 degrees Celsius/350 degrees Fahrenheit. Grease 10 muffin liners and line a 12-count muffin tin with them.
2. Combine the butter, sugar, salt, vanilla extract, and eggs in a large mixing basin. After that, add the milk and stir until everything is well blended.
3. Sift the coconut flour and baking powder together in a separate bowl. Stir together the wet and dry ingredients until well blended.
4. Fill the ten muffin pans about three-quarters full with batter. Bake the cupcakes on the middle rack for seventeen-twenty minutes, or until a skewer inserted in the center comes out clean.
5. Allow ten minutes for the cupcakes to cool in the oven before transferring to a wire rack to cool completely. Frost after it has cooled.

KETO RED VELVET CAKE

Prep Time: 5 Minutes

Cook Time: 25 Minutes

Serves: 12

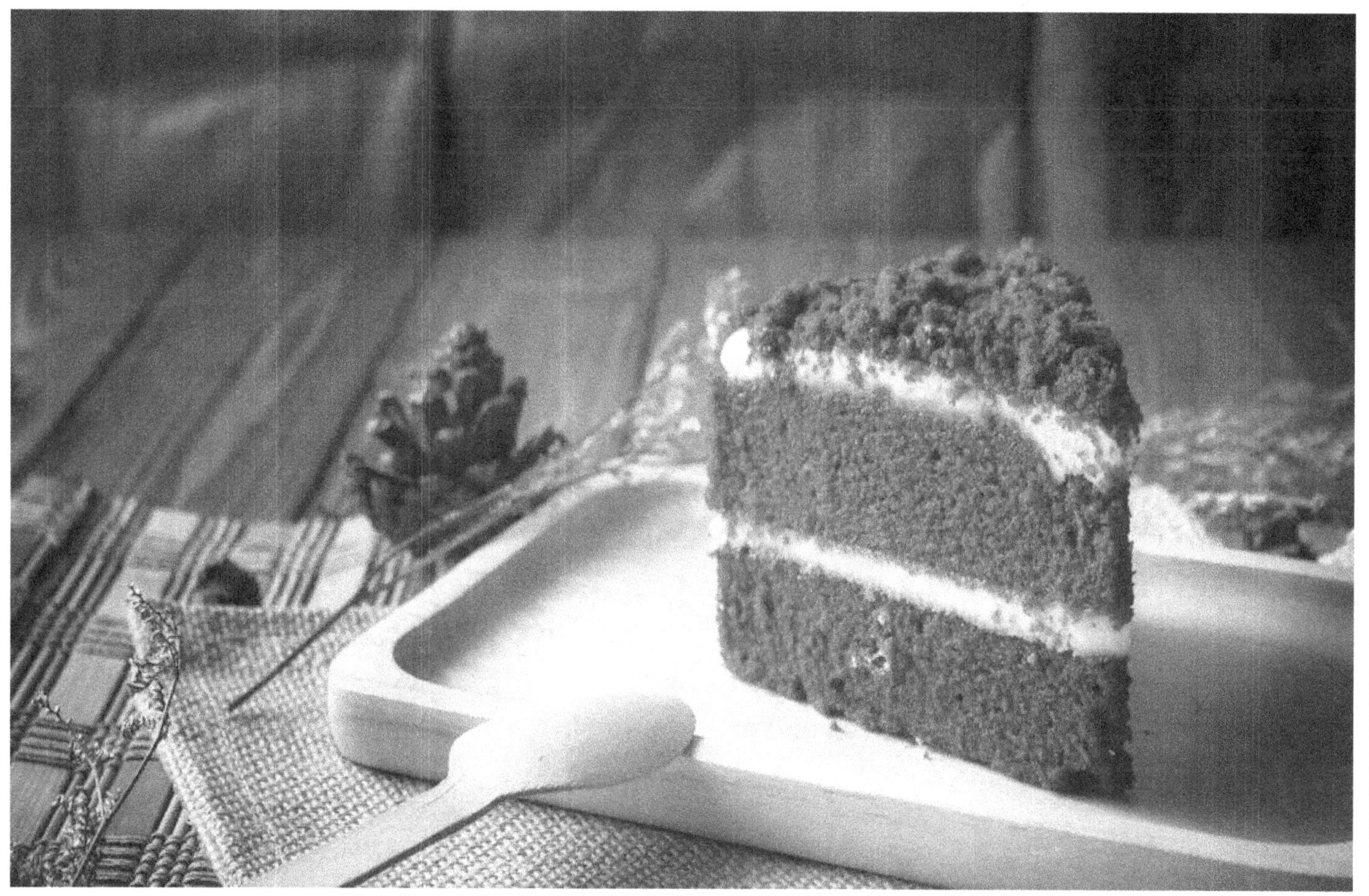

This low-carb red velvet cake is delicious and fluffy, with a low-carb cream cheese icing on top! It only requires 6 key ingredients and can be prepared in just one dish in less than 25 minutes

Nutrition

Calories: 167kcal | Carbohydrates: 4g | Protein: 6g | Fiber: 2g | Fat: 16g

Net Carbohydrates: 2g | Sodium: 113mg

Ingredients

- 4 large eggs room temperature
- 1/2 cup granulated sweetener of choice monk fruit sweetener or erythritol
- 2 cups almond flour blanched almond flour
- 2 tablespoon coconut oil softened
- 1 cup cream cheese frosting
- 1-2 drops red food coloring
- 1 teaspoon baking powder
- 1 teaspoon vanilla extract
- 1/4 teaspoon salt
- 1 teaspoon butter extract optional

Instructions

1. Preheat the oven to 180 degrees Celsius/350 degrees Fahrenheit. Set aside a 9-inch cake pan that has been sprayed with cooking spray.
2. Combine your dry ingredients in a small mixing dish. Whisk together your eggs, sweetener, coconut oil, vanilla extract, and butter extract in a separate dish until well blended. Fill in the blanks using red food coloring.
3. Gently stir the dry ingredients into the wet until everything is well blended. Place the batter in a prepared cake pan and bake for twenty-five to twenty-seven minutes, or until a skewer inserted in the center comes out clean.
4. Remove the cake from the oven and cool thoroughly before icing.

CRUNCHY KETO BERRY MOUSSE

Prep Time: 10 Minutes

Cook Time: 0 Minutes

Chill Time: 4 Hours

Serves: 8

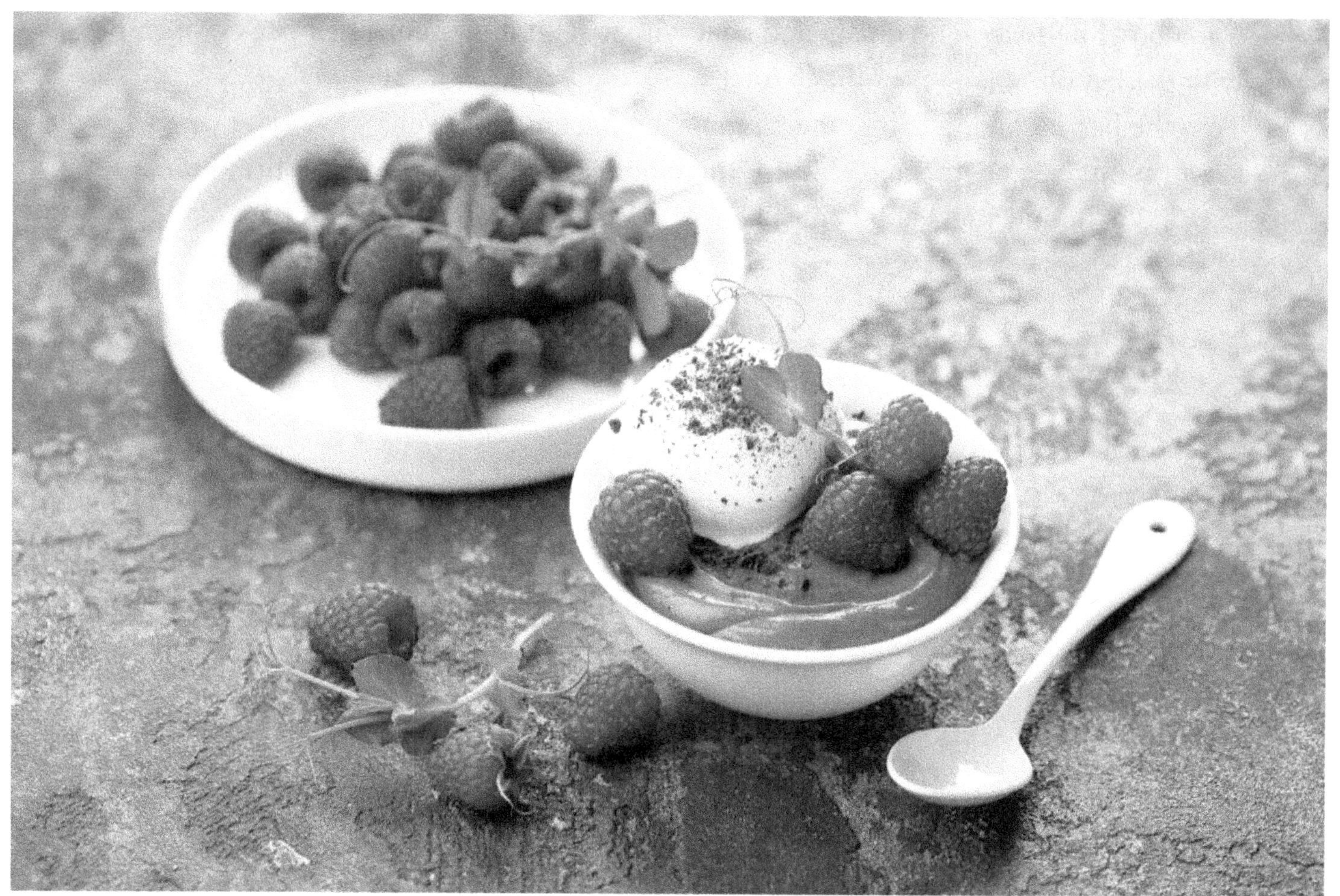

Whip up amazing tastiness with this creamy, creative mousse. It's keto and so simple to make that any cook can throw it together in the afternoon and wow everyone after dinner. With berries in the mix, plus the crunch of pecans and a touch of lemon zest, everyone gathered at your table will appreciate the festive treat

Nutrition

Calories: 256kcal | Protein: 2g | Fat: 26g | Net Carbohydrates: 3g

Ingredients

- 2/3 cup fresh raspberries or fresh strawberries or fresh blueberries
- 2 oz. chopped pecans
- ½ lemon, the zest
- ¼ teaspoon vanilla extract
- 2 cups heavy whipping cream

Instructions

1. Fill a bowl halfway with cream and beat with a hand mixer until soft peaks form. Finish with the lemon zest and vanilla extract.
2. Toss the berries and nuts into the whipped cream and mix well.
3. Cover with plastic wrap and chill for three hours or more to achieve a firm mousse.
4. If you don't mind a less solid consistency, you can eat the dessert right away.

HOMEMADE KETO BOUNTY BARS

Prep Time: 5 Minutes

Cook Time: 5 Minutes

Serves: 24

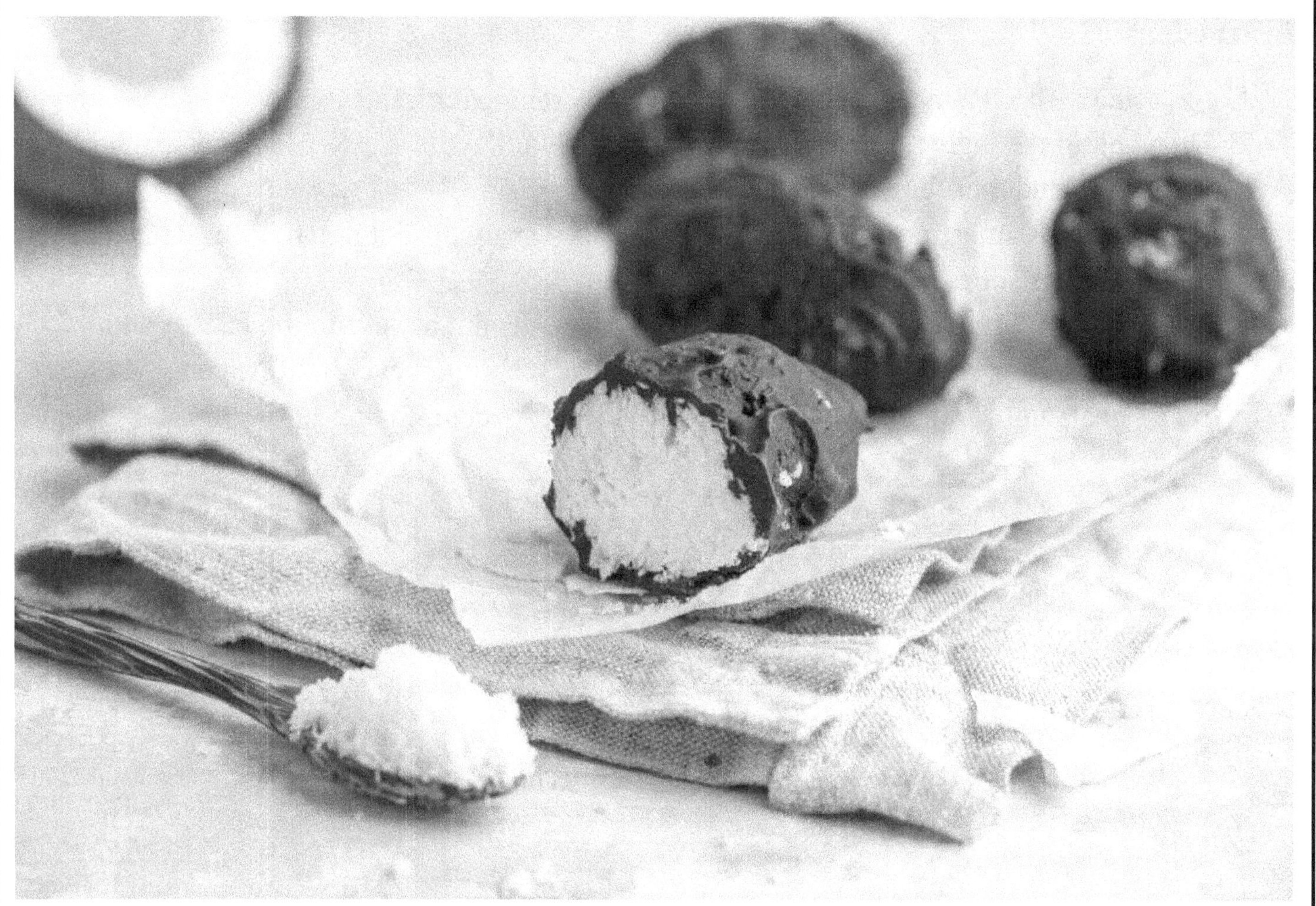

A keto-friendly version of a simple candy bar recipe for homemade bounty bars! These homemade bounty bars, also known as mounds bars, are super low carb and sugar-free and only take 5 minutes to make! Gluten-free, Paleo, Vegan.

Nutrition

Calories: 168kcal | Carbohydrates: 8g | Fiber: 5g | Net Carbohydrates: 3g | Protein: 3g

Fat: 13g

Ingredients

- 4 cups unsweetened shredded coconut
- 2/3 cup canned coconut milk
- 2-3 cups chocolate chips of choice
- 2/3 cup coconut oil, melted
- 1/4 cup keto maple syrup

Instructions

1. Set aside a 10 x 10-inch square pan lined with parchment paper.
2. Blend all of the ingredients, except the chocolate, until a thick batter remains in a high-powered blender or food processor, or big mixing dish.
3. Pour the coconut batter into the prepared pan and firmly push it down. Refrigerate until the mixture is solid.
4. Melt your preferred chocolate chips. Remove the coconut bars from the freezer and immediately dip each one in the melted chocolate, coating it evenly. Refrigerate the bounty bars until solid once all of the chocolate has been used up.

KETO CHOCOLATE BARK

Prep Time: 3 Minutes

Cook Time: 1 Minute

Chill Time: 30 Minutes

Serves: 12

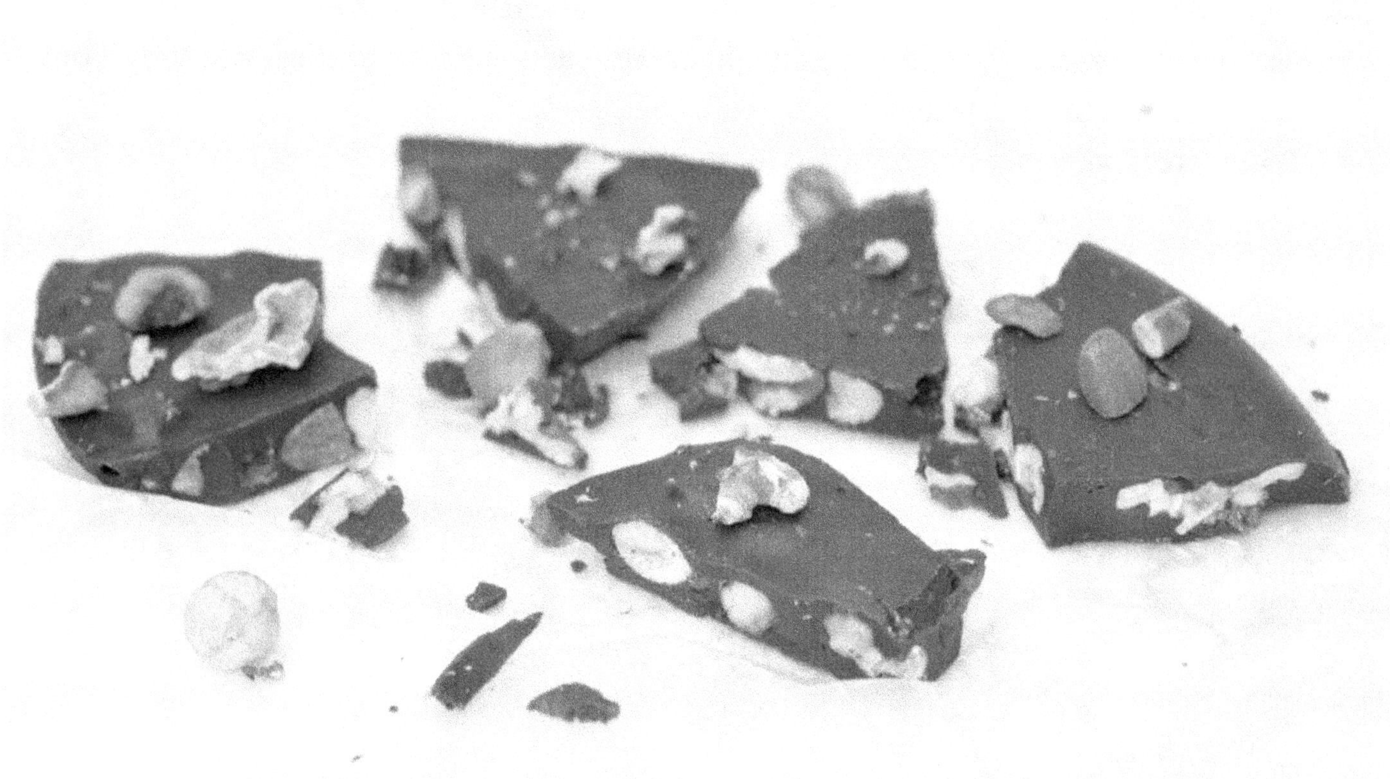

This keto bark has only two ingredients and is packed with crispy almonds. In addition, this chocolate almond bark is dairy-free and sugar-free, and it just takes a few minutes to make.

Nutrition

Calories: 174kcal | Carbohydrates: 8g | Protein: 3g | Fat: 17g | Fiber: 5g

Net Carbohydrates: 3g | Sodium: 1mg

Ingredients

- 1/2 cup roasted almonds unsalted
- 2 cups chocolate chopped
- 1/4 teaspoon flaky sea salt optional

Instructions

1. Set aside a large baking sheet lined with parchment paper. Place the almonds in a large mixing bowl and set aside.
2. Add your chocolate to a microwave-safe bowl or a small saucepan. Microwave for thirty seconds at a time, stirring after each until mostly melted. Whisk everything together until it's smooth and glossy.
3. Pour the melted chocolate over the toasted almonds and stir until they are evenly distributed. Transfer the chocolate/almond mixture to the prepared sheet and spread out evenly using a rubber spatula.
4. Before breaking up into pieces, chill for thirty minutes.

KETO CRUNCH BROWNIES

Prep Time: 35 Minutes

Cook Time: 0 Minutes

Chill Time: 4 Hours

Serves: 12

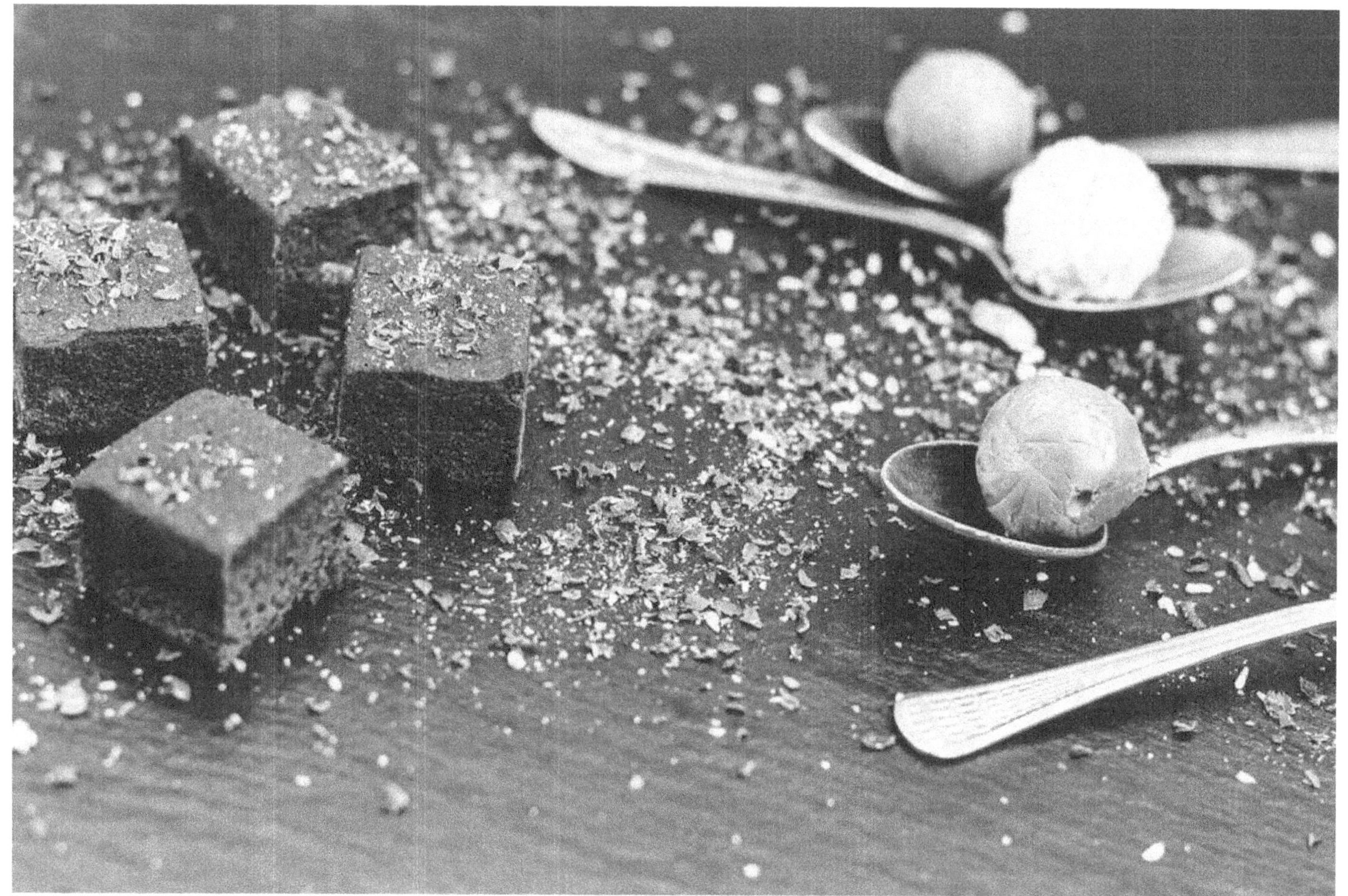

Crunch Brownies are made with a thick, fudgy brownie foundation and a chocolate rice Krispie bar on top! They're impressive and delicious, plus they can be made keto or vegan totally.

Nutrition

Calories: 235kcal | Carbohydrates: 8g | Fiber: 5g | Protein: 6g | Fat: 21g

Net Carbohydrates: 3g | Sodium: 3mg

Ingredients

<u>Keto Crunch Brownies</u>

- 1 batch keto crunch bars
- 1 batch keto brownies

<u>Vegan Crunch Brownies</u>

- 1 batch crunch bars
- 1 batch vegan brownies

Instructions

1. Make your brownies according to the package directions. Allow it cool completely before refrigerating while working on the crunch layer.
2. Make your crunch bars according to the directions. First, remove the brownie base from the refrigerator and, using a rubber spatula, immediately distribute the crunch bar mixture over the top and spread out evenly.
3. To firm up, refrigerate for at least an hour.

KETO COCONUT ICE CREAM

Prep Time: 5 Minutes

Cook Time: 55 Minutes

Chill Time: 3 Hours

Serves: 10

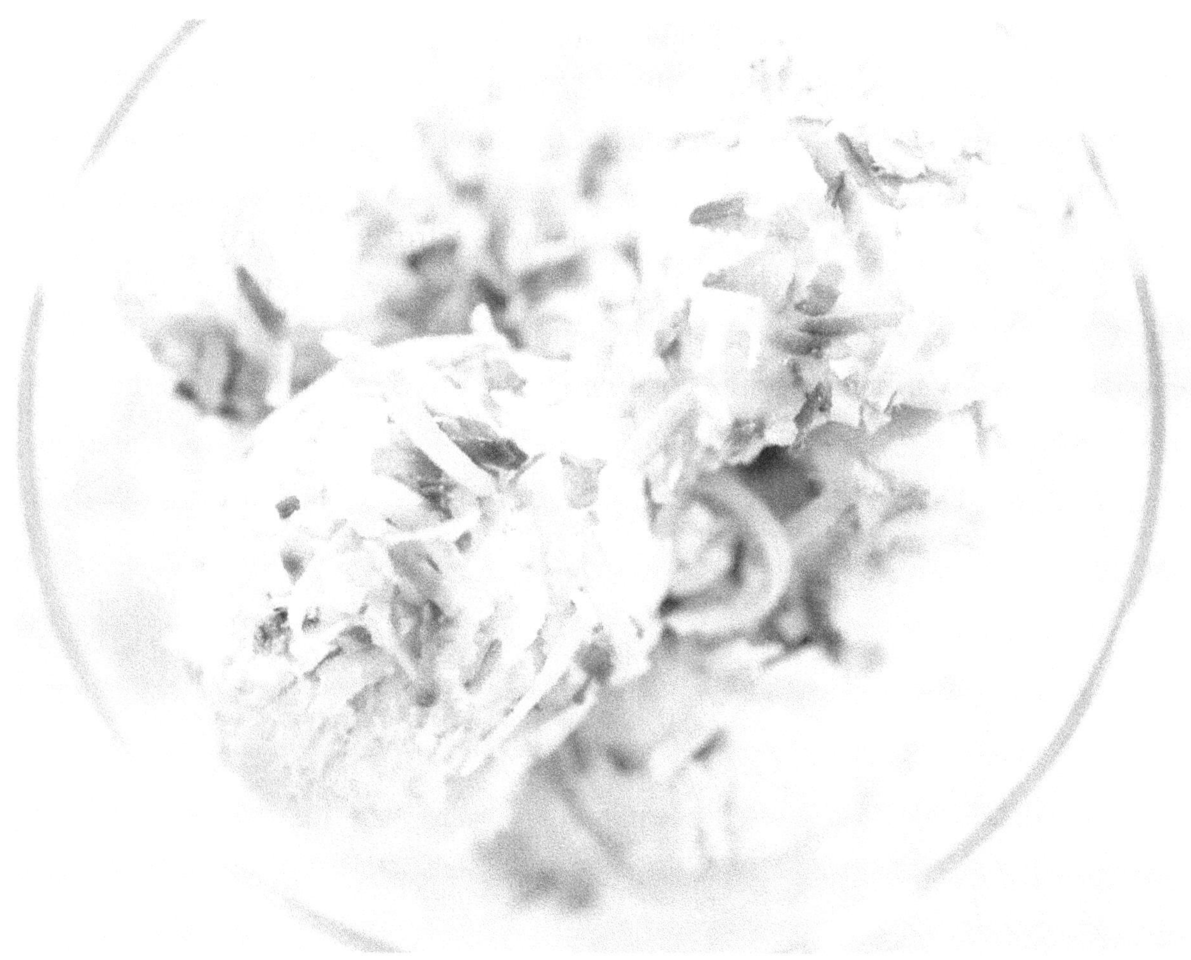

A simple keto and low-carb coconut milk recipe. Only 3 components are needed to make ice cream. It's dairy-free and sugar-free, but you'd never know because it's smooth, creamy, and ready in minutes. There's no need for an ice cream machine because it's no-churn.

Nutrition

Calories: 119kcal | Carbohydrates: 4g | Fiber: 2g | Protein: 4g | Fat: 11g

Net Carbohydrates: 2g | Sodium: 2mg | Potassium: 140mg

Ingredients

- 1/2 teaspoon coconut extract
- 1 13.5 oz can coconut milk chilled
- 1/4 cup keto maple syrup can substitute for pure maple syrup
- 3/4 cup smooth almond butter or cashew butter can sub for any nut
- 1 tablespoon coconut flakes Optional

Instructions

1. Place in the freezer a freezer-friendly container or loaf pan.
2. Combine all of the ingredients in a food processor or high-powered blender and pulse until smooth and creamy. Scrape down the edges of the bowl frequently to ensure the mixture is properly blended.
3. Place the coconut ice cream mixture in the freezer in the pre-frozen container. Stir the ice cream mixture every fifteen minutes for the first hour before allowing it to freeze entirely. Allow at least three hours for the ice cream to freeze.
4. Allow twenty-five to thirty minutes for the coconut ice cream to melt before scooping into bowls with a slightly wet ice cream scoop.
5. Enjoy with a sprinkle of coconut flakes on top.

KETO CHOCOLATE ICE CREAM

Prep Time: 5 Minutes

Cook Time: 2 Minutes

Chill Time: 2 Hours

Serves: 12

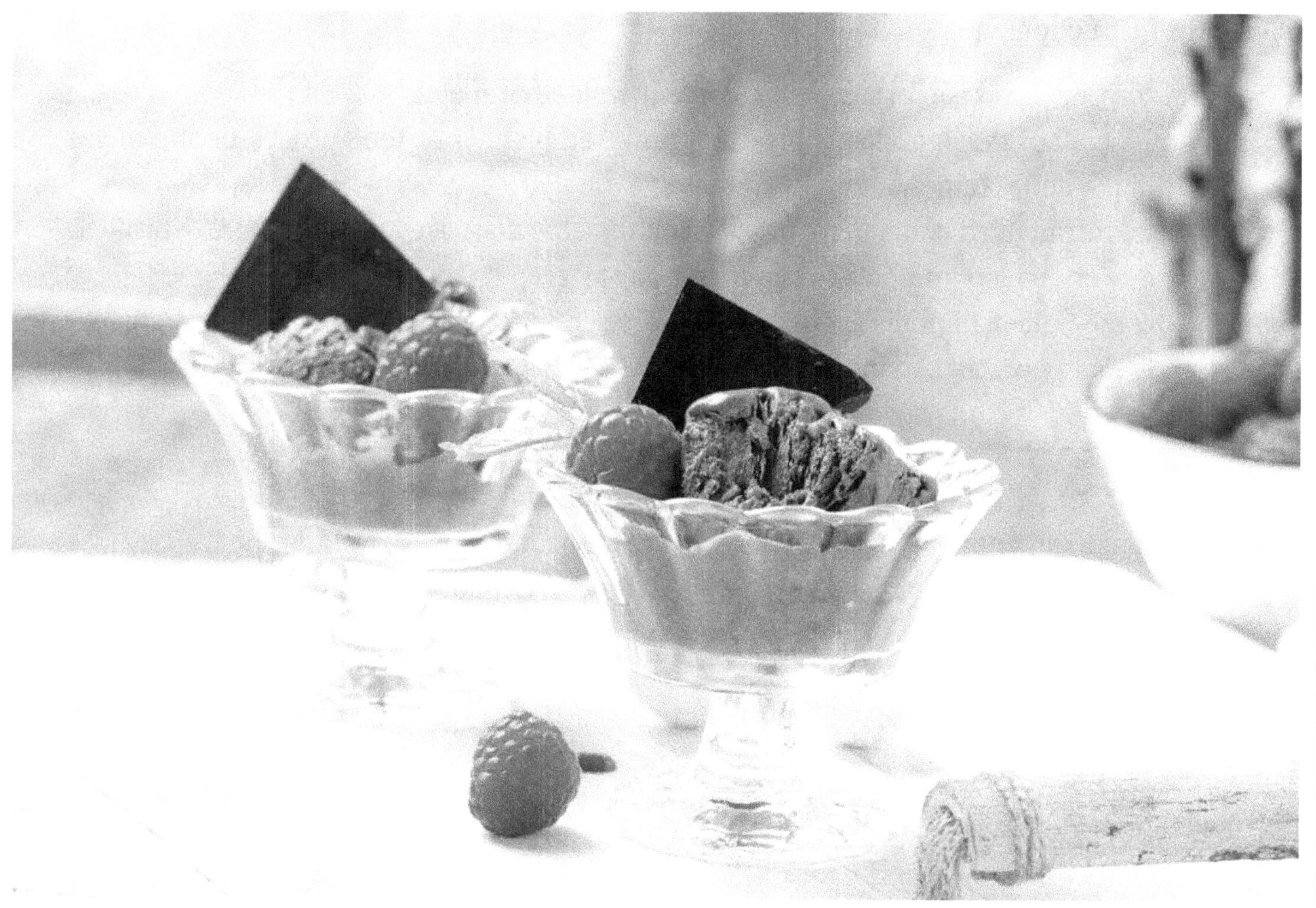

A simple four-ingredient recipe for smooth and creamy keto chocolate ice cream without the need for cream or sugar! This quick homemade ice cream requires no churning or the use of an ice cream maker and is low carb, dairy-free, paleo, and the best chocolate fix.

Nutrition

Calories: 197kcal | Carbohydrates: 5g | Fiber: 4g | Protein: 7g | Fat: 18g

Net Carbohydrates: 1g | Sodium: 3mg

Ingredients

- 1.5 cups almond butter can sub for any nut or seed butter
- 2 13.5 oz can full-fat coconut milk chilled
- 1/4 cup neutral alcoholic spirit of choice
- 2 servings chocolate stevia
- 5 tablespoon cocoa powder

Instructions

No-Churn Instructions

1. Freeze your bread pan or ice cream container made of metal.
2. Combine all of the ingredients in a high-powered blender or food processor and blend until thick and creamy.
3. Fill the refrigerated container halfway with the chocolate ice cream mixture. Stir the liquid every twenty minutes for the first hour to keep it from freezing solid.
4. Allow ten-fifteen minutes for thawing before scooping out. Before serving ice cream, lightly dampen your scoop.

Ice Cream Maker Instructions

1. Freeze your ice cream container that is made of metal.
2. Blend until smooth in a high-powered blender or food processor. Pour the ice cream mixture into the cold pan and set aside for forty-five minutes to harden up somewhat. If your freezer has room, you can also put your blender in there.

KETO CHOCOLATE PUDDING

Prep Time: 10 Minutes

Cook Time: 5 Minutes

Serves: 12

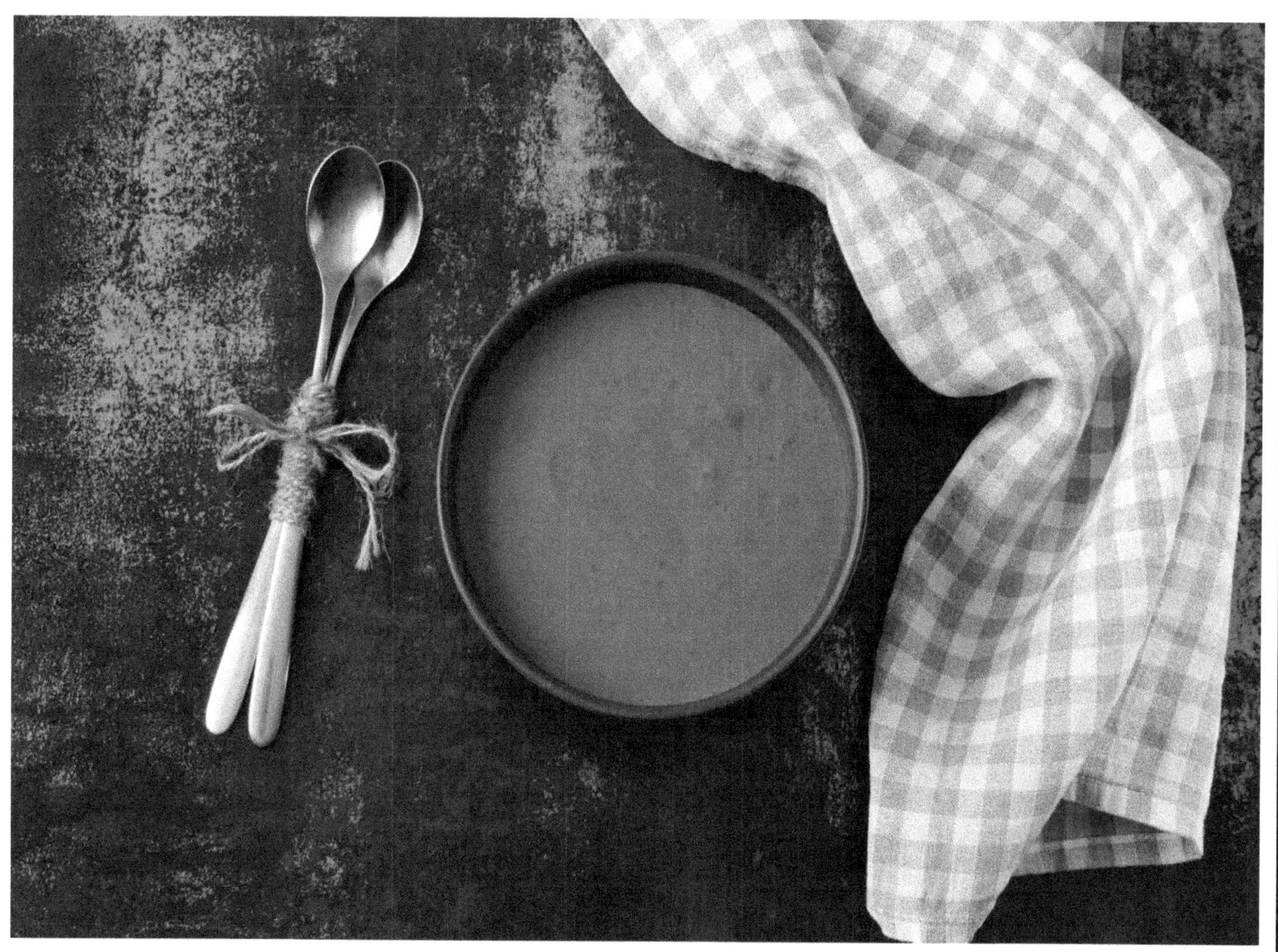

You won't believe how rich and creamy this keto chocolate pudding is when you learn it's created with only 5 ingredients! In addition, this keto pudding is low in Carbohydrates and sugar-free, making it ideal for serving as a sophisticated dessert.

Nutrition

Calories: 194kcal | Carbohydrates: 8g | Fiber: 5g | Protein: 5g | Fat: 19g

Net Carbohydrates: 3g | Sodium: 113mg | Potassium: 62mg

Ingredients

- 3/4 cup granulated sweetener of choice monk fruit sweetener or erythritol
- 1/3 cup cornstarch Can use xanthan gum
- 2 cups chocolate chopped
- 1/2 cup heavy cream
- 1/2 cup cocoa powder
- 4 cups milk of choice

Instructions

1. Cover an 8×4-inch loaf pan with parchment paper and grease it. Set aside.
2. Whisk together all of your ingredients, except the chocolate, in a large mixing bowl.
3. Place the mixture in a saucepan over low heat after straining it. Stir it regularly for two to three minutes once it starts to simmer. Add the chopped chocolate and continue to cook for another two minutes, or until the chocolate melts.
4. Remove the pudding mixture from the heat and stir until the chocolate has completely melted. Pour the mixture into the prepared loaf pan through a strainer. Refrigerate for at least six hours or overnight.
5. Invert the pudding upside down onto a large plate or serving dish after carefully removing it from the loaf pan. Remove the parchment paper from the pudding and sprinkle it with chocolate powder. Slice and serve right away.

KETO LEMON MERINGUE PIE

Prep Time: 10 Minutes

Cook Time: 5 Minutes

Serves: 8

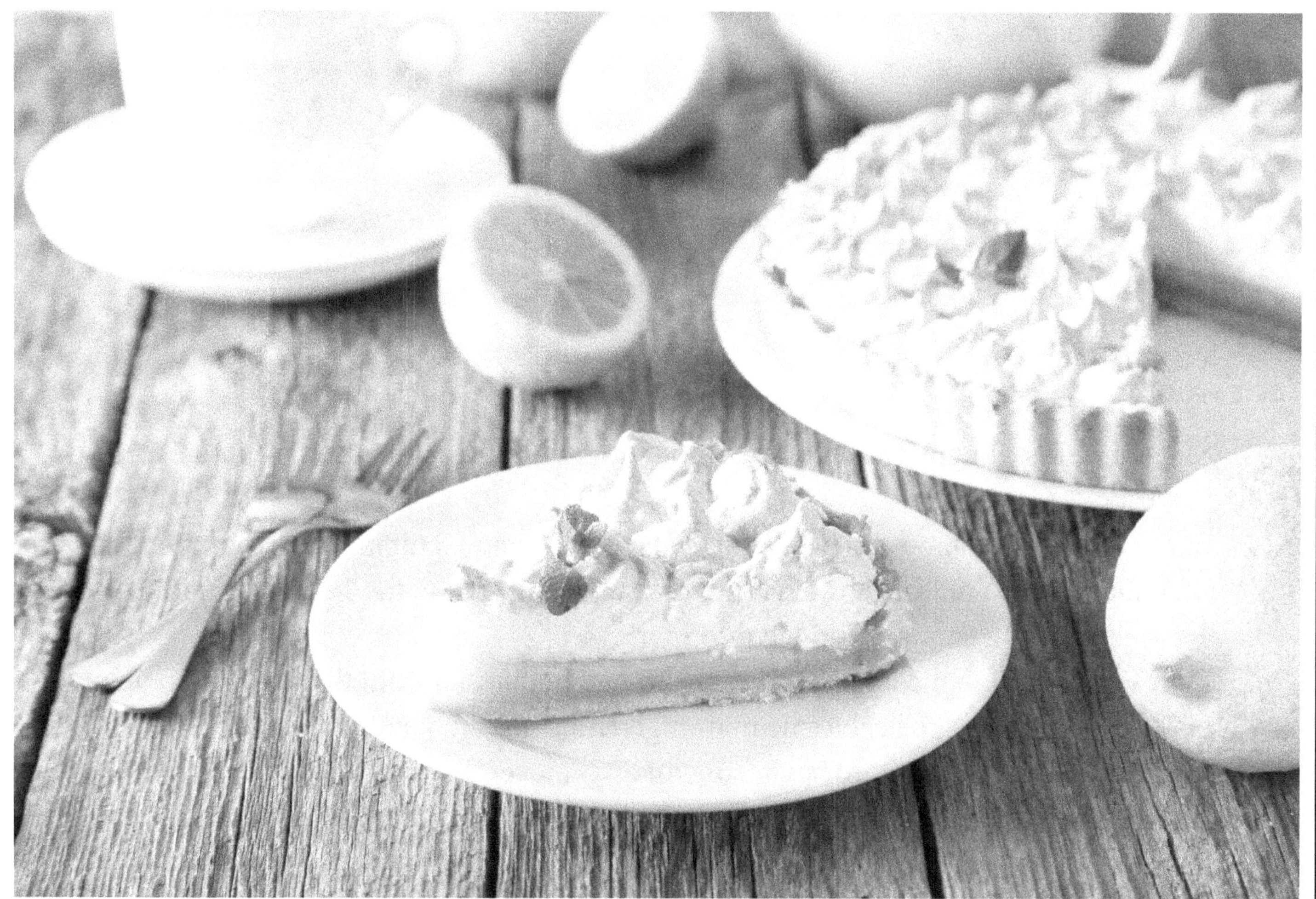

The perfect keto lemon meringue pie- A delectable vegan lemon curd with vegan meringue on top! This vegan + keto lemon pie is a show-stopper because it contains no processed sugar or eggs.

Nutrition

Calories: 149kcal | Carbohydrates: 16g | Net Carbohydrates: 6g | Fiber: 10g | Protein: 1g

Fat: 1g | Sodium: 1mg | Potassium: 54mg

Ingredients

- 1 9-inch pie crust of choice

For the lemon curd

- 1 cup super-fine sugar caster sugar
- 1/4 teaspoon yellow food coloring
- 1/3 cup corn flour cornstarch
- 1 cup coconut milk
- 3/4 cup lemon juice

For the meringue

- 1/2 cup Aquafaba liquid from 1 x 400 gram can of chickpea water
- 1 cup powdered sugar or sugar-free powdered sugar
- 1/2 teaspoon cream of tartar

Instructions

1. Make the crust for your pie. You can use a store-bought, homemade, or no-bake crust. Set aside.
2. In a saucepan, combine corn flour and super-fine sugar. Combine the lemon juice and coconut milk in a mixing bowl. Slowly drizzle in the yellow food coloring until it's lovely and yellow like a lemon meringue pie color.
3. Increase the heat to medium. Stir for one to two minutes or until the sugar is completely dissolved. Increase the heat to medium-high and cook, frequently stirring, for about five minutes, or until the mixture begins to boil and thicken.
4. Remove the lemon curd from the heat and set it aside. Transfer the lemon curd into the pie shell as fast as possible. To firm up, refrigerate for at least two hours.
5. Start making your vegan meringue once the lemon curd has firmed up. Add your aquafaba to a large mixing bowl and whisk until soft peaks form about five minutes. Continue to beat in the cream of tartar until it is completely mixed. Slowly drizzle in the powdered sugar and beat until stiff, glossy peaks form. Finally, add the vanilla extract to the mixture.
6. Spread the vegan meringue over the top of the lemon pie with a rubber spatula. Brown the tops of the meringue with such a blow torch.

KETO SHORTBREAD COOKIES

Prep Time: 5 Minutes

Cook Time: 15 Minutes

Serves: 12

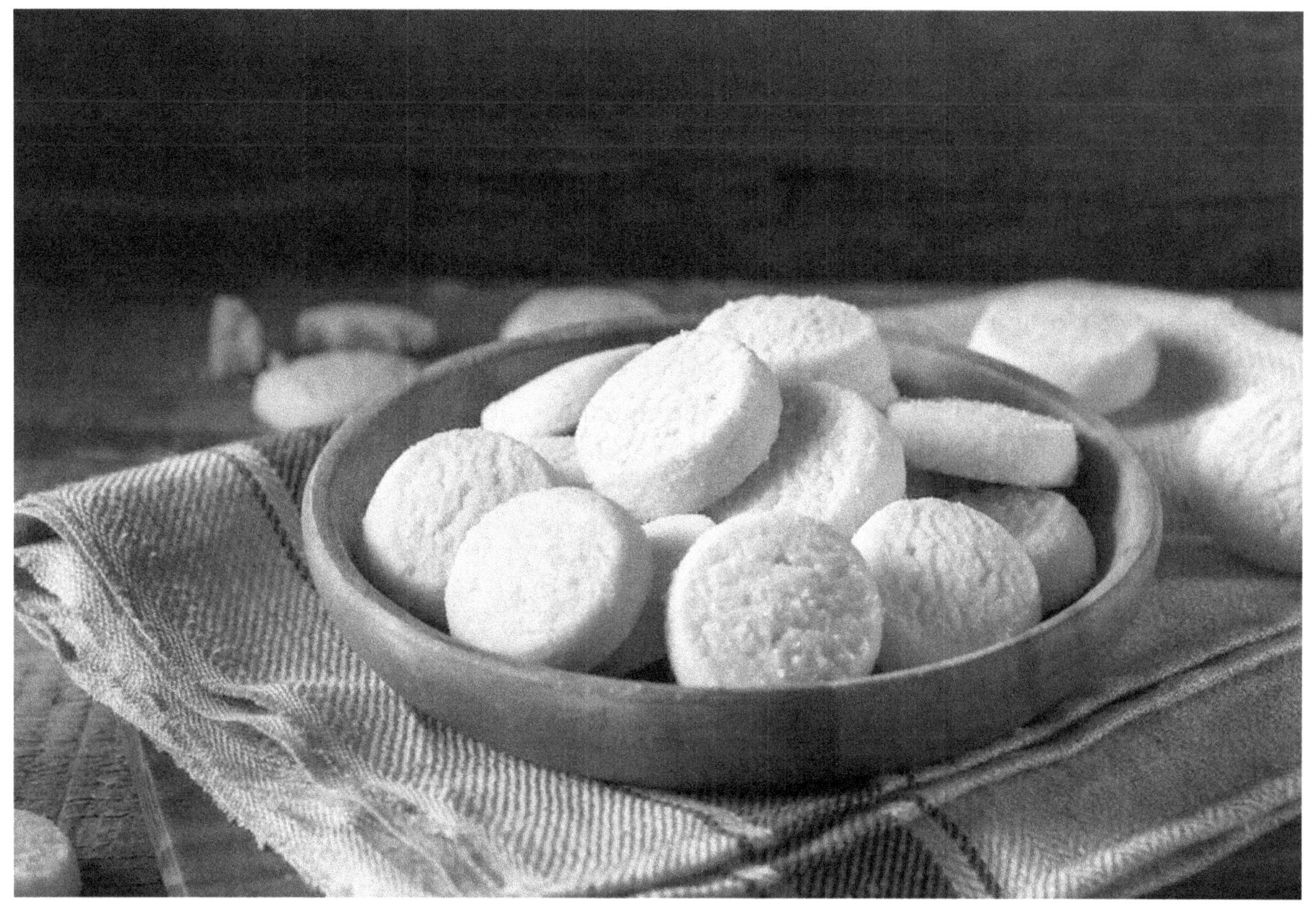

These keto shortbread cookies are a low-carb version of conventional shortbread. Cookies that are crumbly and buttery, created with only 5 ingredients and no grains or sugar.

Nutrition

Calories: 152kcal | Carbohydrates: 4g | Net Carbohydrates: 2g | Protein: 5g Fiber: 2g

Fat: 14g | Sodium: 46mg | Potassium: 12mg

Ingredients

- 2 large eggs room temperature
- 1 teaspoon vanilla extract
- 3/4 cup granulated sweetener of choice erythritol or monk fruit sweetener
- 2 cups almond flour blanched almond flour
- 1/4 cup butter softened and salted

Instructions

1. Preheat the oven to 180 degrees Celsius/350 degrees Fahrenheit. Using parchment paper, line a large baking sheet.
2. Combine the softened butter and granulated sweetener in a large mixing basin. Combine all ingredients in a hand mixer and beat until smooth. Add the vanilla essence and eggs one at a time, mixing well after each addition. Finally, gently mix in the almond flour until everything is well blended.
3. Form 12-15 dough balls with a big spoon or cookie scoop and place them on the prepared baking sheet. Each ball should be pressed into a cookie shape, then crossed with a fork on both sides.
4. Bake the cookies for seventeen-twenty minutes, or until the edges start to turn brown. Remove the cookies from the oven and set them aside to cool completely.

KETO OREO COOKIES

Prep Time: 5 Minutes

Cook Time: 12 Minutes

Serves: 12

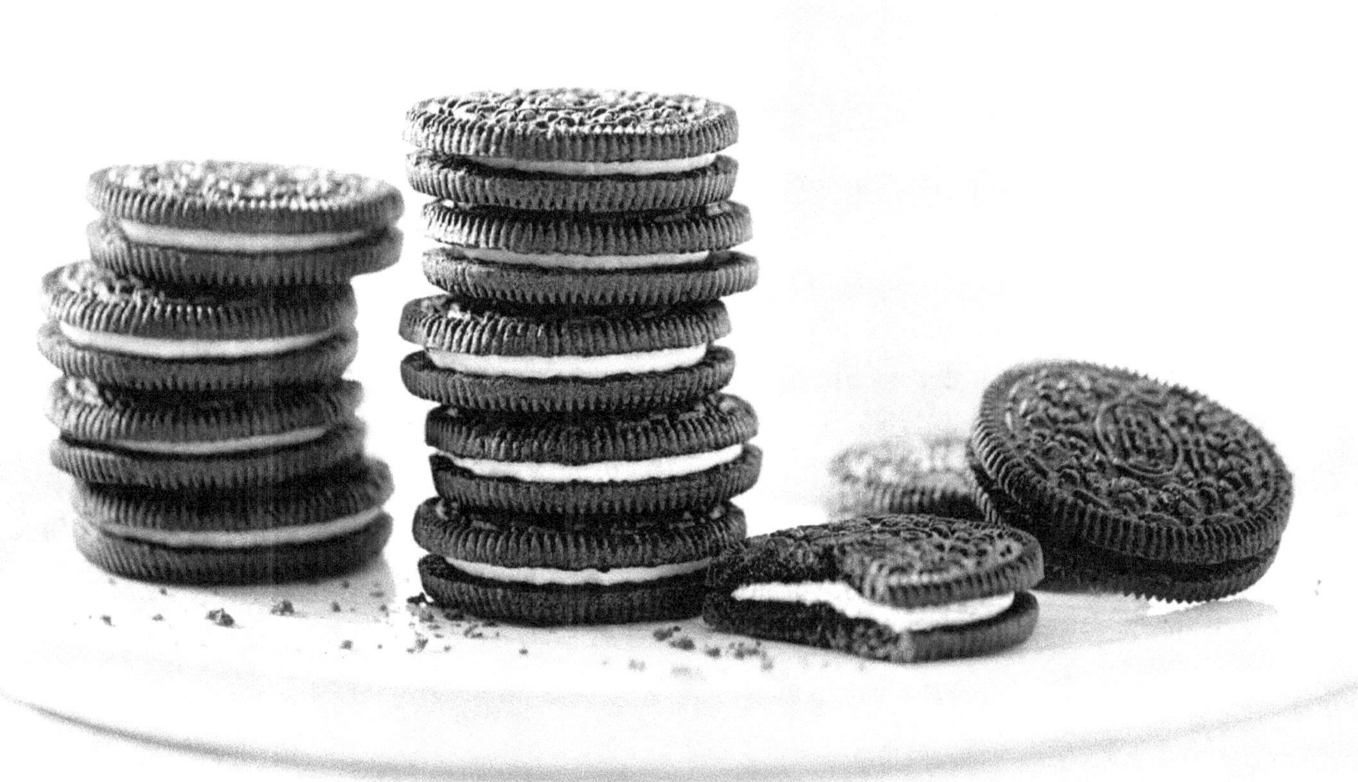

Keto Oreos are a low-carb version of the popular Oreo cookies. This Keto Oreo cookie recipe is quick and easy to create, with a sugar-free vanilla cream filling.

Nutrition

Calories: 194kcal | Carbohydrates: 10g | Fiber: 7g | Protein: 6g | Fat: 14g

Net Carbohydrates: 3g | Sodium: 236mg

Ingredients

- 6 large eggs room temperature
- 2/3 cup granulated sweetener of choice
- 2 cups keto vanilla frosting
- 1/2 cup cocoa powder
- 1/2 teaspoon baking soda
- 1/2 cup almond flour
- 1/2 cup butter softened
- 1 1/2 cups coconut flour
- 1 teaspoon vanilla extract
- 1/4 teaspoon salt

Instructions

1. Preheat the oven to 180 degrees Celsius. Set aside two large baking pans lined with parchment paper.
2. Combine the almond flour, coconut flour, cocoa powder, baking soda, and salt in a large mixing bowl. Mix thoroughly. In a separate bowl, whisk together the granulated sugar, eggs, and butter until creamy. Finally, add the vanilla extract to the mixture.
3. Mix together your wet and dry ingredients until a thick dough form. Form 24 tiny dough balls using your hands. Place the dough on the two baking trays and form it into cookies.
4. Bake the cookies for twelve minutes before removing them from the oven and allowing them to cool completely on the baking pans after the cookies have cooled, spread icing on half of them, and press down with the remaining cookies.

NO-BAKE COOKIES AND CREAM CHEESECAKE (KETO)

Prep Time: 5 Minutes

Cook Time: 0 Minutes

Chill Time: 4-6 Hours

Serves: 12

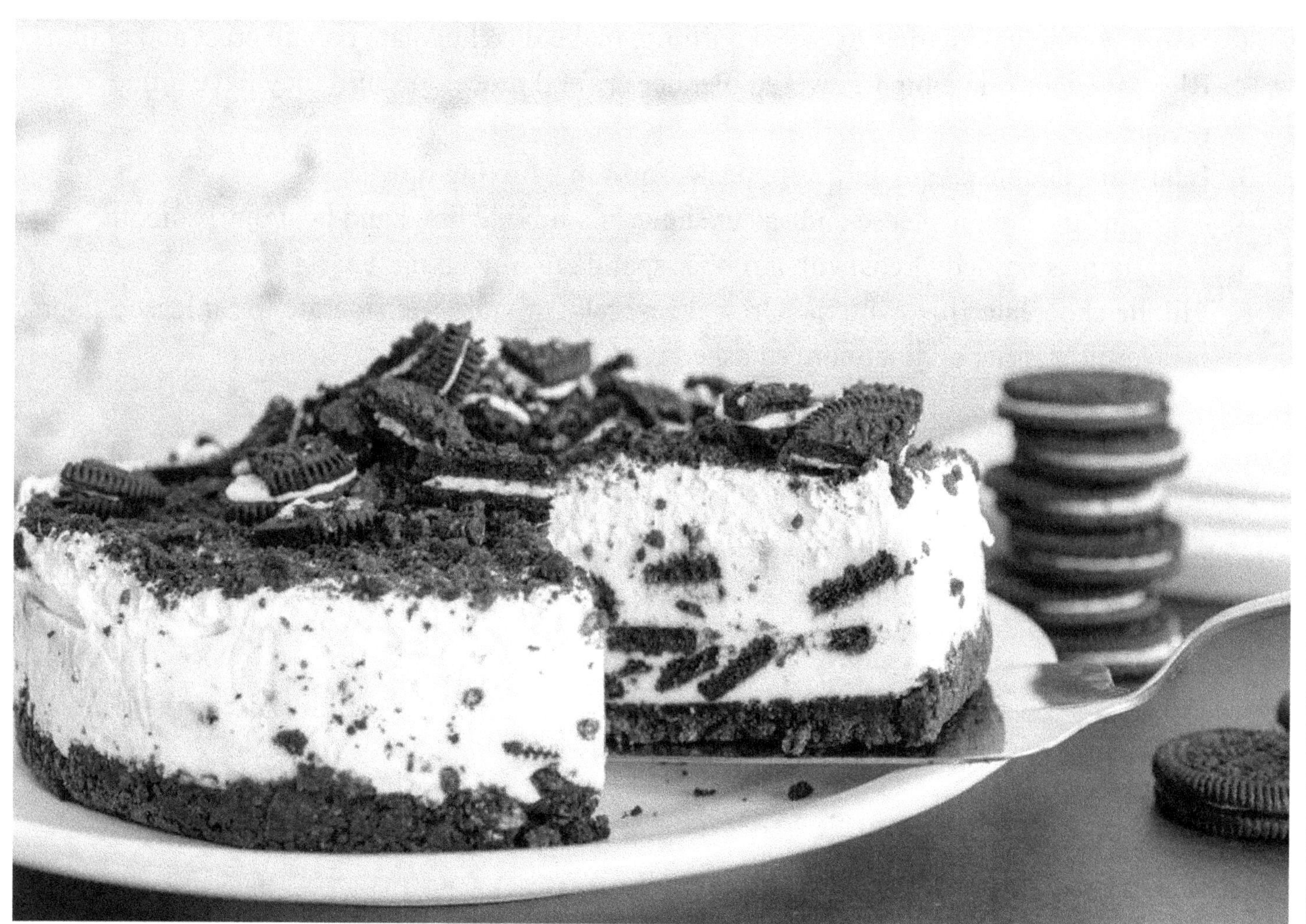

The iconic Oreo Cheesecake gets a keto and low carb makeover with No-Bake Cookies and Cream Cheesecake! This Oreo Cheesecake is a show-stopping keto dessert with only 5 ingredients and a handmade cookie crust.

Nutrition

Calories: 149kcal | Net Carbohydrates: 1g | Carbohydrates: 3g Fiber: 2g | Protein: 2g

Fat: 14g| Sodium: 69mg | Potassium: 41mg

Ingredients

- 1 cup heavy cream
- 12 Homemade Oreo Cookies
- 1/2 cup sweetener of choice
- 1 chocolate cookie crust
- 8 ounces cream cheese

Instructions

1. While you're making the cheesecake filling, make the chocolate cookie crust and chill it.
2. Blend the Oreos in a high-powered blender or food processor until they have a fine texture.
3. Beat your double cream until firm peaks form in a mixing bowl.
4. Combine the cream cheese and caster sugar in a mixing bowl and beat until smooth.
5. Fold in the smashed Oreos with a rubber spatula until well mixed.
6. Fill the chocolate crust with the Oreo cheesecake mixture. Refrigerate for at least 6 hours, or overnight, after adding more smashed cookies.

KETO BLONDIES

Prep Time: 5 Minutes

Cook Time: 20 Minutes

Serves: 12

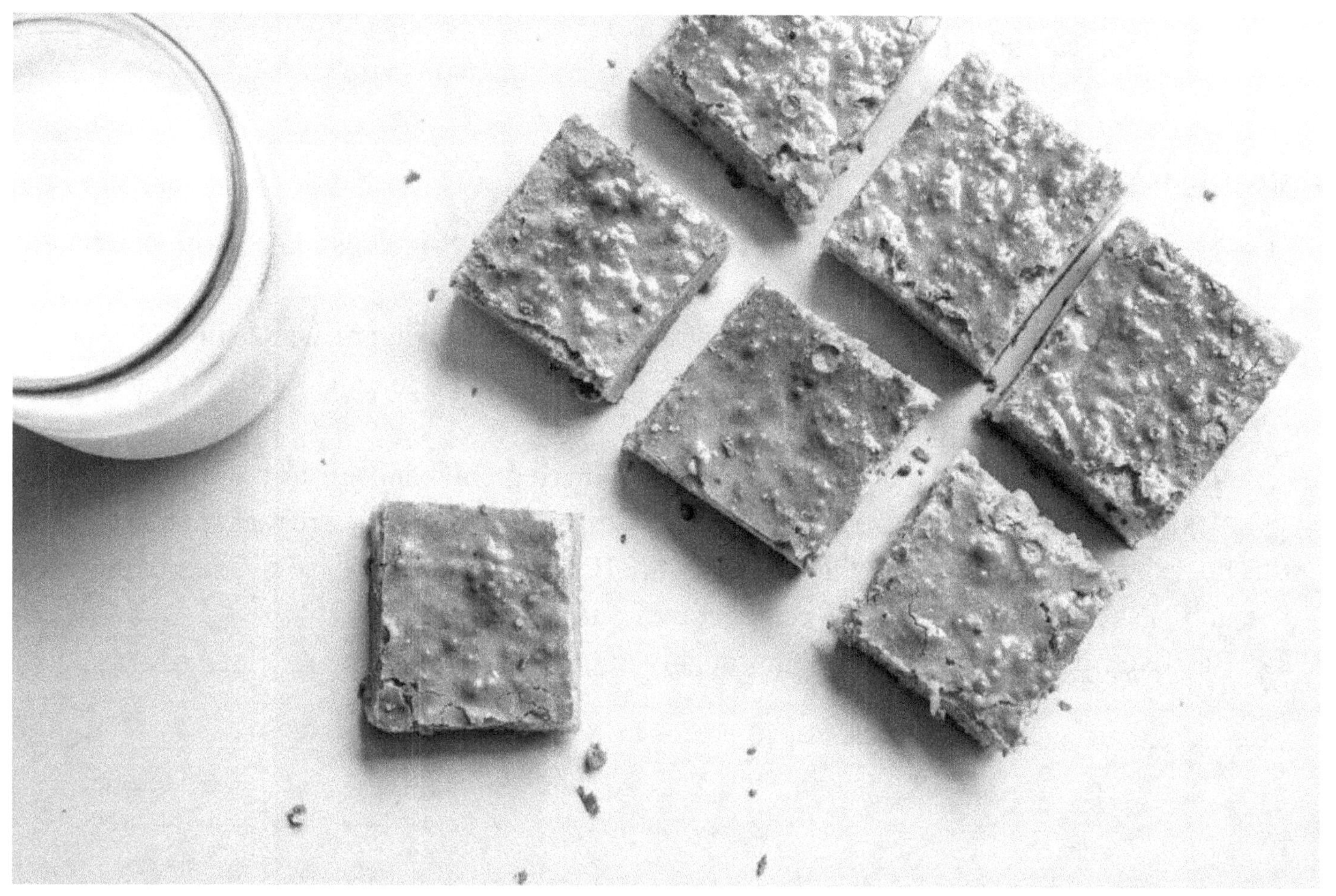

Keto blondies cooked in under 20 minutes are the best keto dessert recipe! Almond flour blondies that are fudgy and done in 20 minutes

Nutrition

Calories: 190kcal | Net Carbohydrates: 3g | Carbohydrates: 5g | Protein: 5g | Fiber: 2g

Fat: 18g | Sodium: 124mg | Potassium: 12mg

Ingredients

- 2 large eggs
- 1/2 cup butter or dairy-free butter, softened
- 1/2 cup mix-ins nuts, seeds, chocolate chunks, etc.
- 1 cup golden monk fruit sweetener
- 1/2 cup keto chocolate chips
- 2 cups almond flour
- 1 teaspoon baking powder
- 1 teaspoon vanilla extract

Instructions

1. Preheat the oven to 180 degrees Celsius. Set aside an 8 x 8-inch pan lined with parchment paper.
2. Combine the almond flour and baking powder in a large mixing dish and stir well. Whisk together the golden monk fruit sweetener, eggs, softened butter, and vanilla extract in a separate bowl until well blended.
3. Now combine the wet and dry ingredients in a mixing bowl and stir just until mixed. Next, fold in your chocolate chips and other desired mix-ins with a rubber spatula.
4. Pour the blondie batter into the prepared pan. Bake for twenty-twenty five minutes, or until a skewer inserted into the center comes out clean.
5. Remove from the oven and cool thoroughly in the pan.

CHOCOLATE TART (KETO)

Prep Time: 5 Minutes

Cook Time: 5 Minutes

Chill Time: 2 Hours

Serves: 12

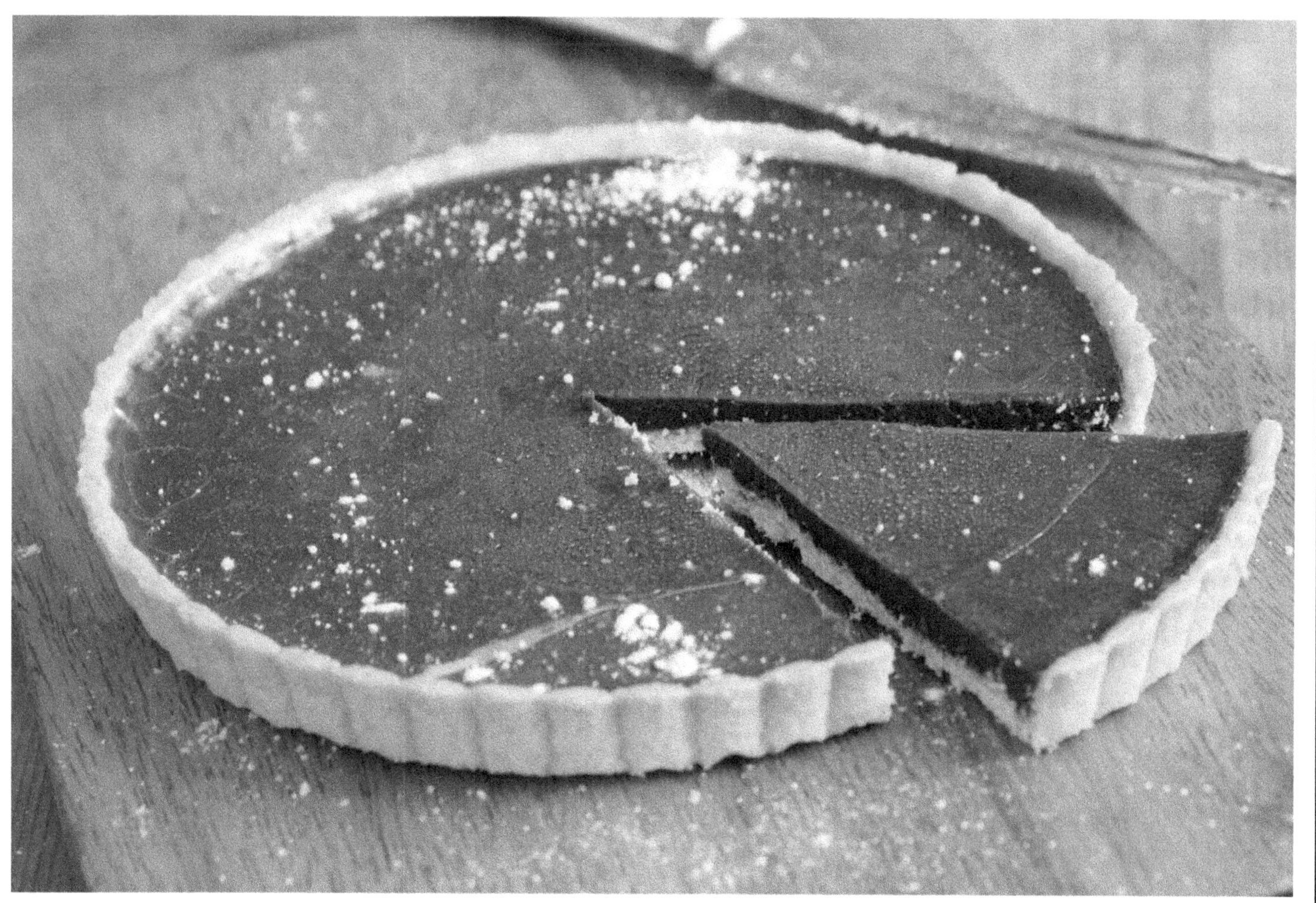

Only 4 ingredients are required to make this simple no-bake chocolate tart. For a smooth, creamy, and rich chocolate tart filling, no dairy or eggs are necessary. It's gluten-free and vegan, and it's simple to make keto and sugar-free.

Nutrition

Calories: 189kcal | Net Carbohydrates: 3g | Carbohydrates: 6g | Fiber: 3g

Protein: 3g | Fat: 16g | Sodium: 4mg | Potassium: 62mg

Ingredients

- 2 cups chocolate chips of choice can use a chopped chocolate bar
- 1 1/2 cups coconut milk canned
- 1 8-inch pie crust of choice, no-bake or baked
- 1 teaspoon vanilla extract

Instructions

1. Make an 8-inch springform pan with your handmade or store-bought pie crust. Set aside.
2. Warm-up your coconut milk in a small saucepan or microwave-safe bowl. When the chocolate/chocolate chips are warm, add them and set them aside for two to three minutes. After that, combine the coconut milk and chocolate in a mixing bowl and whisk until smooth and shiny. Next, add the vanilla extract and whisk to combine.
3. Fill the pie crust with the chocolate tart filling. Refrigerate for at least two hours or until the mixture is solid. If preferred, season with a pinch of salt.

LOW-CARB KETO CHOCOLATE CUPCAKES

Prep Time: 10 Minutes

Cook Time: 20 Minutes

Serves: 10

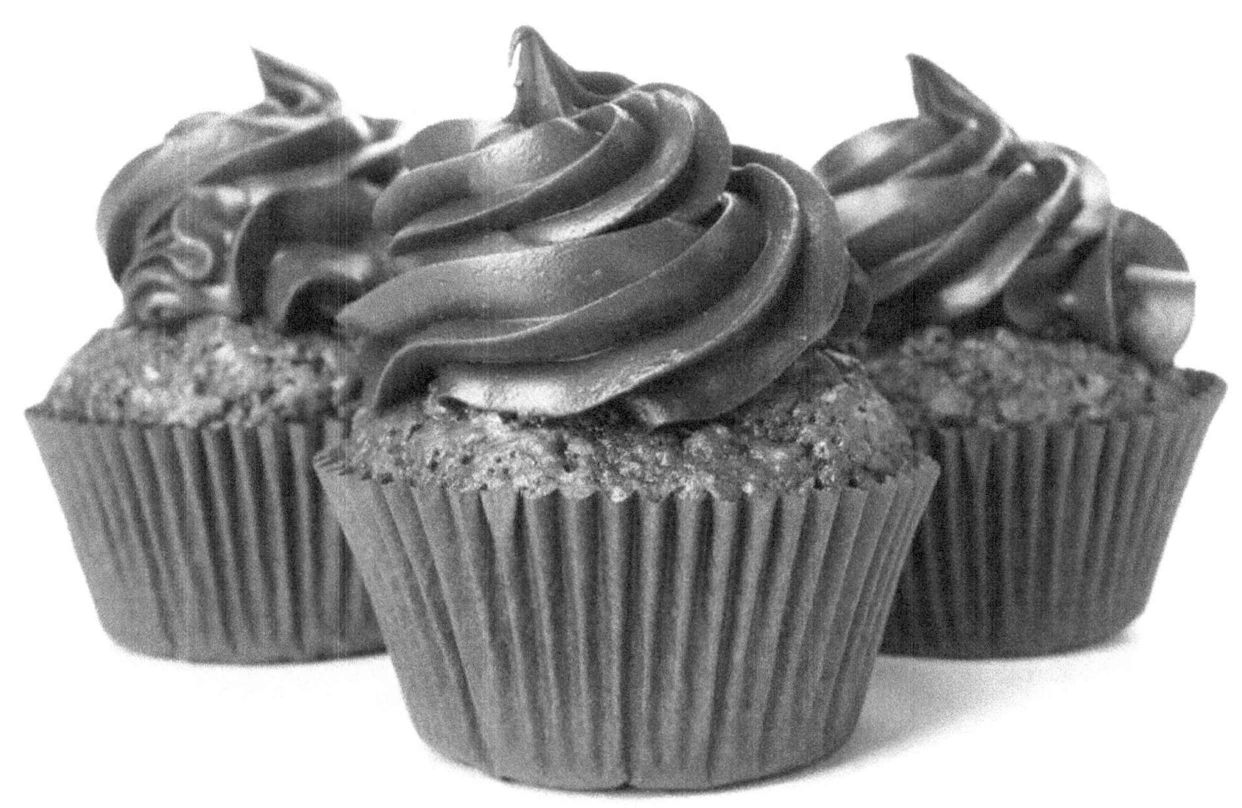

No-sugar keto chocolate cupcakes made with almond flour! This recipe for keto low-carb chocolate cupcakes is rich, sweet, and ready in under 30 minutes.

Nutrition

Calories: 479 | Fat: 48g | Protein: 10g | Fiber: 5g | Sugar: 3g | Total Carbohydrates: 11g

Net Carbohydrates: 6g

Ingredients

- 3 large Eggs
- 1/2 cup Besti Monk Fruit Allulose Blend
- 2 cups Wholesome Yum Blanched Almond Flour
- 1/2 cup unsweetened almond milk
- 1/2 recipe Keto Chocolate Frosting
- 1/3 cup butter softened
- 6 tablespoon Cocoa powder
- 1/2 tablespoon Baking powder
- 1/4 teaspoon Sea salt
- 1 teaspoon Vanilla extract

Instructions

1. Preheat the oven to 350°F. In a muffin tray, line 10 cups with paper liners.
2. Using a hand mixer, cream butter, and sweetener together in a large mixing bowl until frothy.
3. Mix almond flour, cocoa powder, baking powder, and salt in a bowl and mix.
4. In a separate bowl, whisk together the eggs, almond milk, and vanilla extract.
5. Cook for twenty-twenty five minutes, or until a toothpick inserted in the center comes out clean.
6. Allow muffins to cool completely before topping with 2 tablespoons keto chocolate frosting each cupcake.

ALMOND FLOUR KETO BLUEBERRY SCONES

Prep Time: 10 Minutes

Cook Time: 20 Minutes

Serves: 8

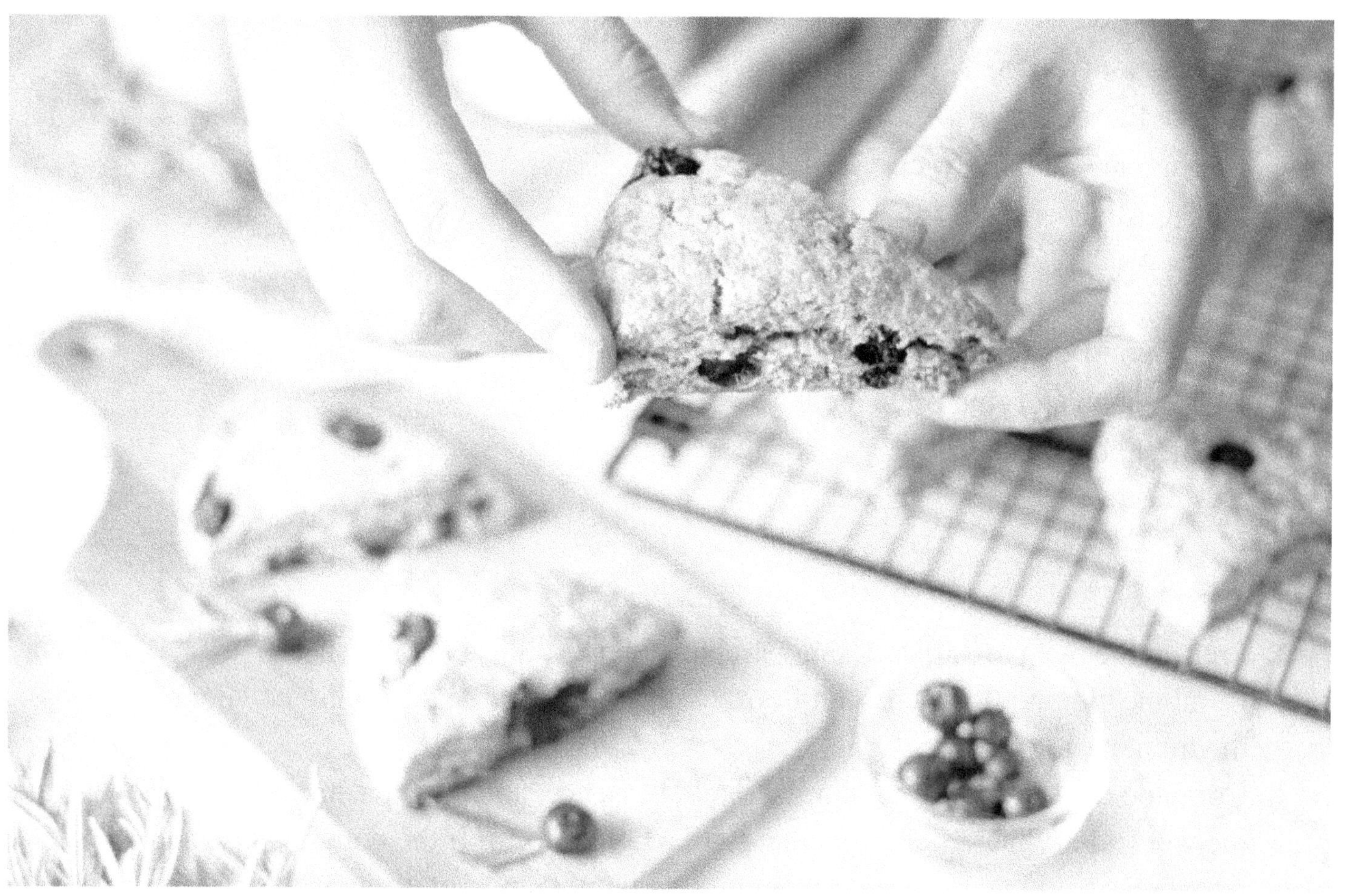

Fresh blueberries abound in these keto almond flour scones! In addition, you'll enjoy these low-carb keto blueberry scones, which have only 4 grams of Carbohydrates and taste just like genuine.

Nutrition

Calories: 159 | Fat: 13g | Protein: 5g | Fiber: 4g | Sugar: 3g | Total Carbohydrates: 8g

Net Carbohydrates: 4g

Ingredients

<u>Scones</u>

- 1/4 cup unsweetened almond milk
- 1 cup Wholesome Yum Blanched Almond Flour
- 1/4 cup Wholesome Yum Coconut Flour
- 2 tablespoon Coconut oil
- 3 tablespoon Besti Erythritol
- 1/2 teaspoon Baking powder
- 1/4 teaspoon Sea salt
- 1 large Egg
- 1 teaspoon vanilla extract
- 1/2 cup Blueberries

<u>Glaze</u>

- 1 teaspoon Besti Powdered Erythritol
- 1 tablespoon Coconut oil melted
- 2 tablespoon Blueberries

Instructions

1. Preheat the oven to 350°F. Using parchment paper, line a baking sheet.
2. Combine almond flour, coconut flour, erythritol, sea salt, and baking powder in a medium mixing bowl.
3. Combine coconut oil, almond milk, vanilla essence, and egg in a small mixing bowl. Fold the wet and dry ingredients together until a dough form. If the dough is dry, add a teaspoon of almond milk at a time until it is flexible but not crumbly or stiff. Toss the blueberries into the dough and fold them in.
4. Form a disc out of the dough in the prepared pan, about 1 inch thick. Cut each wedge into eight pieces. Separate the pieces by about 1 inch. Bake for eighteen to twenty-two minutes, or until golden brown.
5. Prepare the glaze in the meantime. In a blender, puree the glaze ingredients. To capture and discard the blueberry skins, strain through a fine-mesh screen. Drizzle the glaze over the scones once they've finished baking and spread evenly. Allow scones to cool completely before glazing them.

RASPBERRY WHITE CHOCOLATE KETO POPSICLES

Prep Time: 5 Minutes

Cook Time: 5 Minutes

Chill Time: 4 Hours

Serves: 6

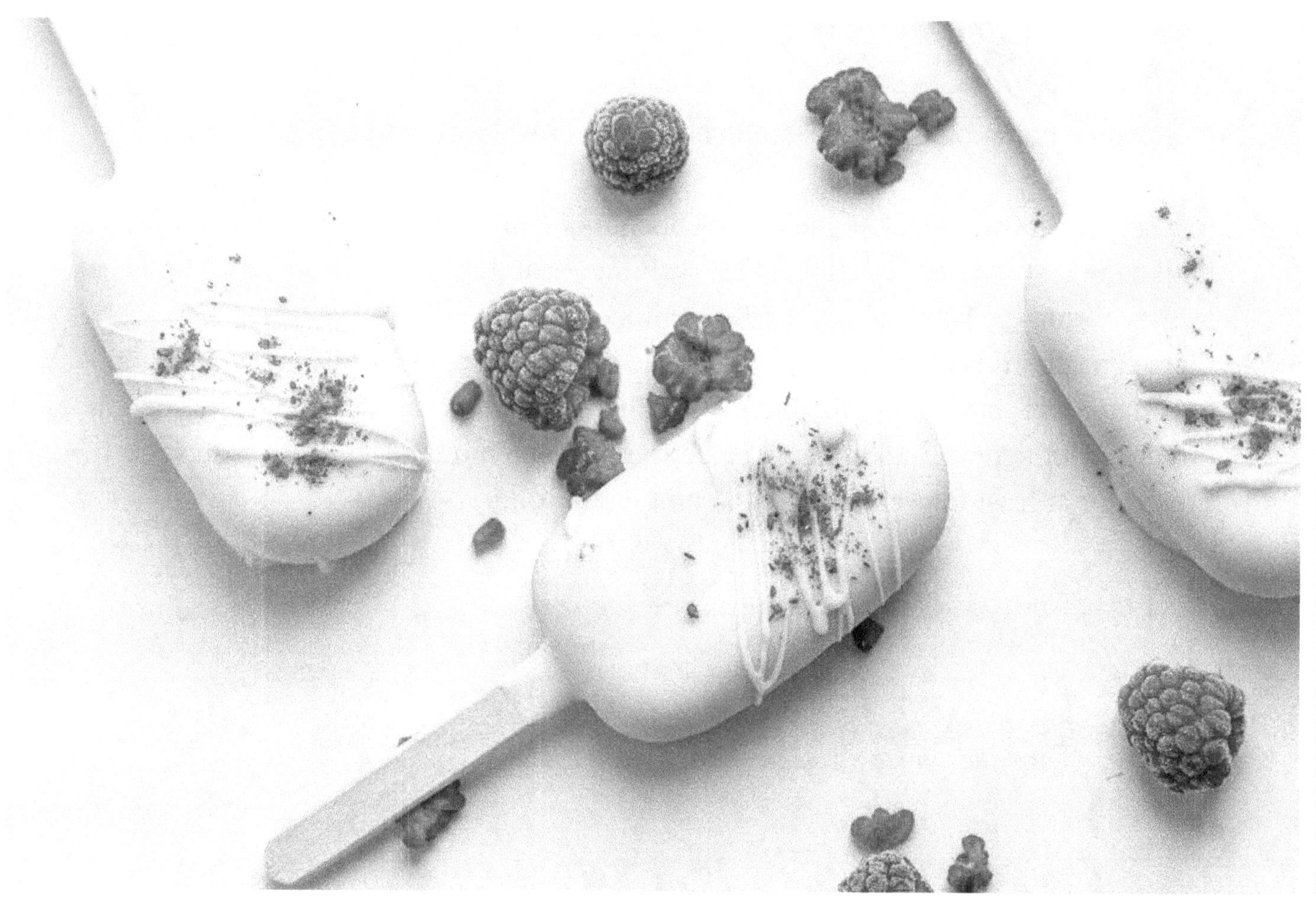

Raspberry white chocolate keto popsicles are made with only 5 ingredients and take only 10 minutes to prepare! Sweet and creamy, these low-carb keto-friendly popsicles have only 3.7g net Carbohydrates each.

Nutrition

Calories: 295 | Fat: 24.8g | Net Carbohydrates: 4.9g | Fiber: 11.2g | Sugar2.4g

Protein: 3.5g | Total Carbohydrates: 12.1g

Ingredients

- 1 cup Raspberries
- 6 Popsicle sticks
- 3/4 cup Choc Zero Sugar-Free White Chocolate Chips
- 1/4 cup Besti Powdered Allulose
- 1 1/4 cups coconut cream
- 1 teaspoon vanilla extract
- 1/4 teaspoon Sea salt

Instructions

1. In a double boiler on the stove, melt chocolate chips. Heat until melted, stirring periodically.
2. In a separate bowl, whisk together the coconut cream, powdered allulose, and sea salt until completely dissolved. If it isn't dissolving, heat it in a double boiler on low heat. Remove from the heat and mix in the vanilla extract.
3. Place 3 raspberries in each of 6 big popsicle molds and pour half of the white chocolate cream mixture into each of the molds. Fill the rest of the way with the white chocolate mixture after adding 3 additional raspberries. In each mold, place a popsicle stick.
4. Freeze for at least four hours or until completely solid.

NO-BAKE FROZEN KETO LOW CARB PEANUT BUTTER PIE

Prep Time: 15 Minutes

Cook Time: 0 Minutes

Chill Time: 2 Hours

Serves: 12

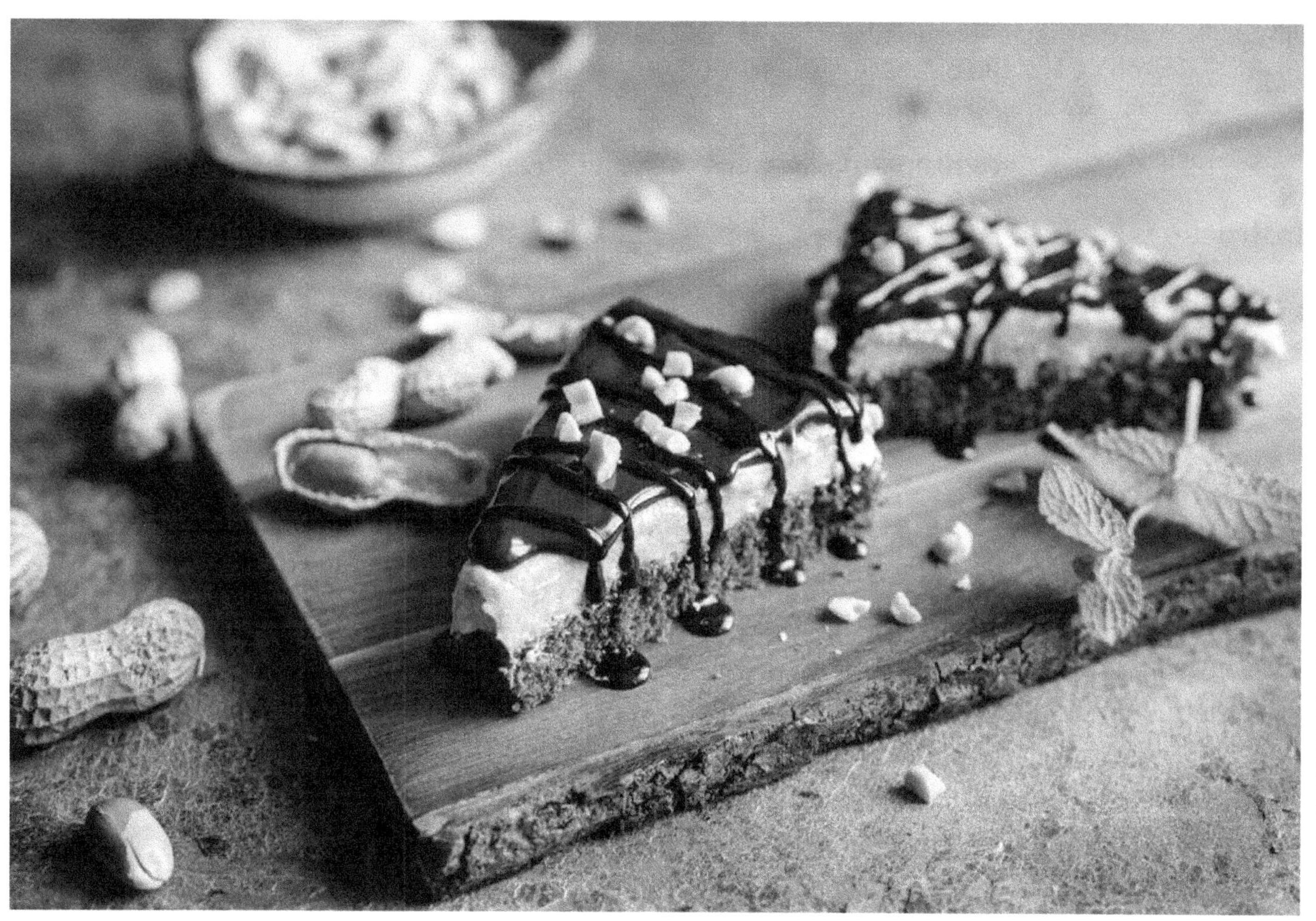

You'll be hooked after you discover how to make keto low-carb peanut butter pie! This rich and delectable no-bake peanut butter pie recipe is sugar-free and easy to make.

Nutrition

Calories: 314 | Fat: 28.7g | Net Carbohydrates: 7.4g | Protein: 7.4g | Fiber: 2.8g

Sugar: 2.4g | Total Carbohydrates: 10.2g

Ingredients

<u>No-Bake Peanut Butter Pie Crust</u>

- 4 medium keto double chocolate cookies
- 6 medium Keto peanut butter cookies
- 2 tablespoons Besti Powdered Allulose
- 1/4 cup butter

<u>Sugar-Free Peanut Butter Pie Filling</u>

- 1 1/8 cups Heavy cream
- 1/3 cup Besti Powdered Allulose
- 3/4 cup Peanut butter
- 1 teaspoon Vanilla extract
- 4 oz Cream cheese softened
- 1 1/8 cups Heavy cream (divided into 6 tablespoon and 3/4 cup)

Instructions

1. In a food processor, combine the cookies. Pulse until the mix resembles crumbs.
2. Pulse in the butter and powdered sweetener until the mixture is homogeneous and crumbly.
3. Refrigerate the dough for approximately fifteen minutes, or until it's less sticky and easier to deal with.
4. To make the crust, press the cookie dough into the bottom and up the sides of a 9-inch pie pan.
5. Place the crust in the freezer for twenty minutes.
6. Meanwhile, whisk together the peanut butter, cream cheese, and powdered sweetener in a large, deep mixing bowl for about 2 minutes, or until frothy. Add the vanilla extract and mix well. Add 1 tablespoon at a time, beat in roughly 6 tablespoons heavy cream until it reaches the consistency of thick frosting.
7. The amount of cream you'll need depends on how thick your peanut butter was, so add 1 tablespoon at a time until it's the consistency of thick icing.
8. 3/4 cup heavy cream, whisked until stiff peaks form in the second bowl. In a large mixing bowl, fold the whipped cream into the peanut butter mixture.
9. Place the filling in the pie pan on top of the crust.
10. Freeze for at least 1 hour or until the mixture is stiff. If it's too firm, immediately out of the freezer, let it sit on the counter for a few minutes to soften, similar to an ice cream cake. Toppings such as melted peanut butter drizzle, melted chocolate drizzle, and more crumbled cookies can be added if desired.

KETO FLAN

Prep Time: 5 Minutes

Cook Time: 45 Minutes

Chill Time: 60 Minutes

Serves: 6

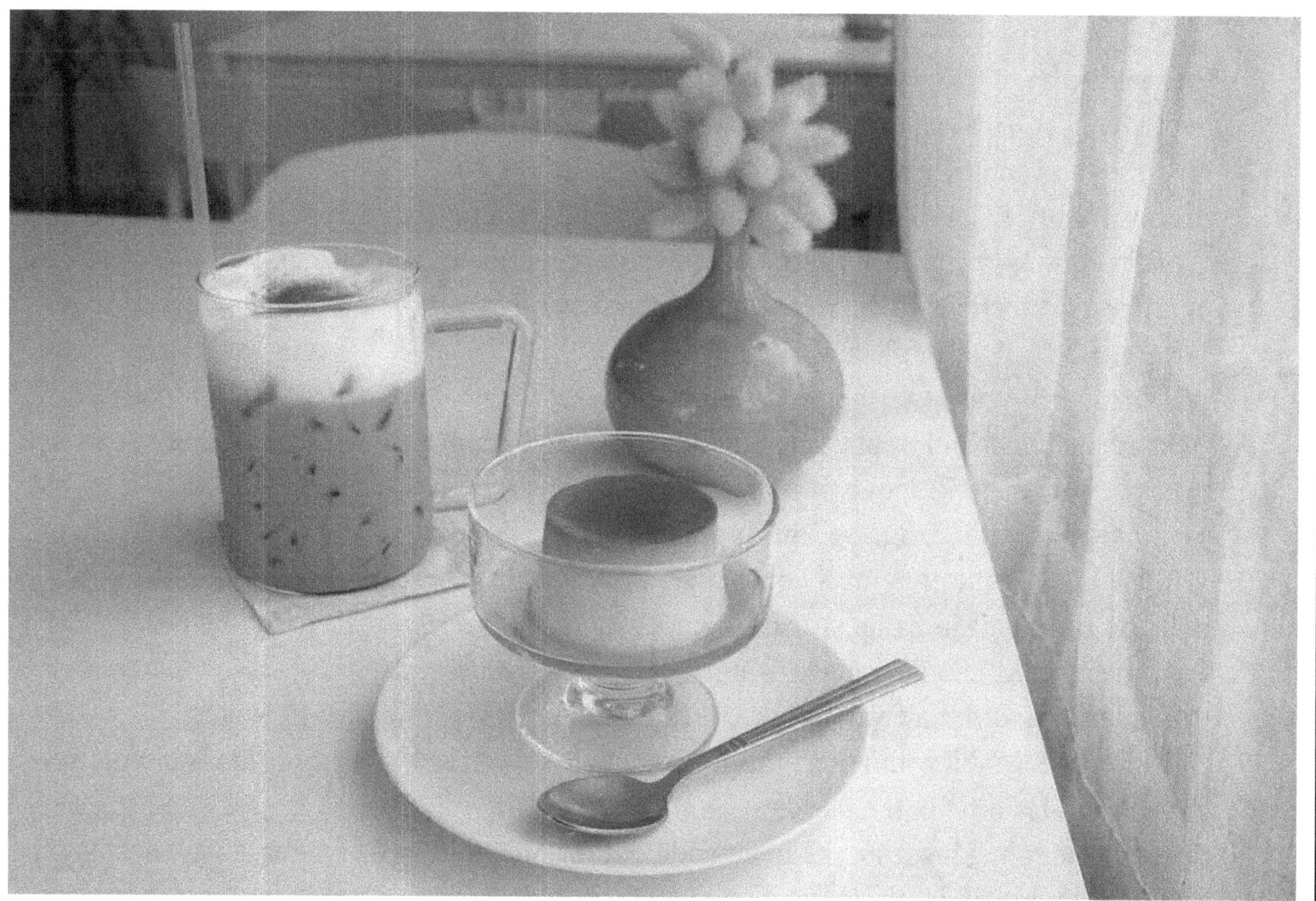

With a vital ingredient for a wonderfully creamy base and burnt caramel on top, this quick low-carb keto flan recipe is amazing. You won't be able to know that this flan is sugar-free.

Nutrition

Calories: 331 | Fat: 33.3g | Protein: 4.8g | Fiber: 0.1g | Sugar: 2.6g

Total Carbohydrates: 2.9g | Net Carbohydrates: 2.8g

Ingredients

- 6 large Egg yolks
- 2 cups Heavy cream
- 2 teaspoon Vanilla extract
- 1 cup Besti Powdered Monk Fruit Allulose Blend
- 1/4 cup Water
- 1 pinch Sea salt

Instructions

1. Preheat the oven to 350°F. Combine 1/2 cup Besti and 1/4 cup water in a small saucepan over low heat. Heat until the sugar is completely dissolved.
2. Increase the heat to bring to a boil, then reduce to low heat and continue to cook for twenty-twenty five minutes, or until a golden syrup form.
3. Working quickly, divide the syrup evenly among 6-ounce ramekins and tilt the ramekins in different directions to distribute the caramel evenly over the bottom and up the edges. In a 9x13 baking dish, place the ramekins.
4. Whisk the egg yolks together in a medium mixing dish.
5. Heat the heavy cream, remaining 1/2 cup Besti, and a pinch of salt in a medium saucepan over medium heat. Remove from heat after bubbles appear around the edges. In a separate bowl, whisk together the vanilla essence and the sugar.
6. While whisking the egg yolks constantly, slowly pour the cream mixture into the bowl with the egg yolks in a thin stream. Tempering is the process of forming the custard.
7. Pour the custard into the ramekins through a fine-mesh sieve.
8. Fill the baking dish halfway up the edges of the ramekins with boiling water.
9. Bake for twenty-thirty minutes, flipping pan halfway through, or until flan is almost set but still jiggles little in the middle.
10. Remove the ramekins from the oven and cool for one hour in the water bath. Then dry the ramekins, put them in plastic wrap, and store them in the refrigerator for up to four days.
11. To serve, run a knife around the outside edges of each ramekin until it begins to spin inside the ramekin.
12. Then, immediately invert a tiny plate with a raised rim on top. Shake the plate up and down until you hear the flan release from the ramekin onto the plate. Lift the ramekin slowly.

SUGAR-FREE KETO MARSHMALLOWS

Prep Time: 15 Minutes

Cook Time: 5 Minutes

Serves: 16

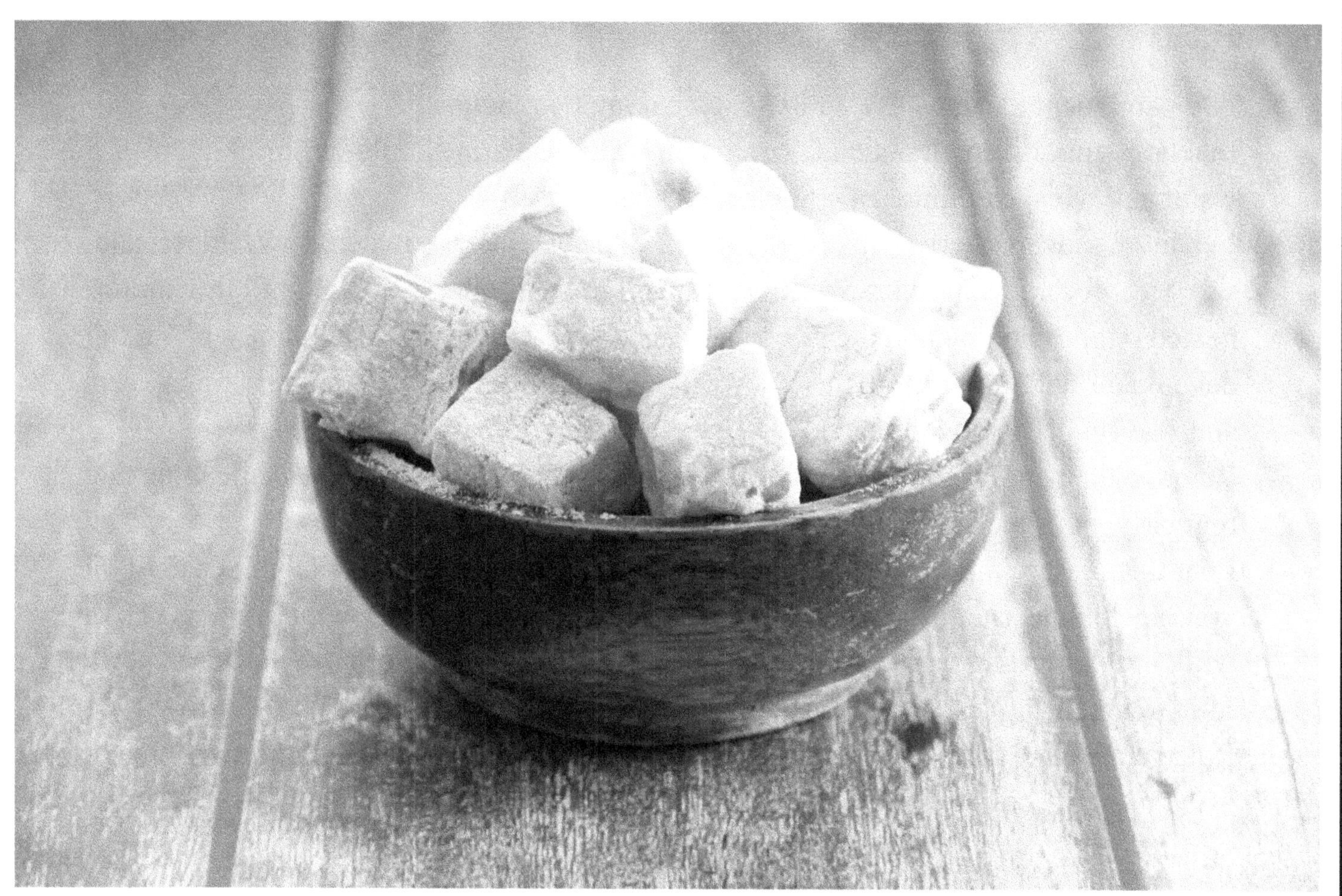

With only three ingredients, you can make sugar-free marshmallows in no time! Without the sugar or corn syrup, these low-carb keto marshmallows have the same flavor and texture you adore.

Nutrition

Calories: 4 | Fat: 0.1g | Protein: 0.7g | Total Carbohydrates: 0.1g | Fiber: 0g

Sugar: 0.1g | Net Carbohydrates: 0.1g

Ingredients

- 1 1/2 cups Besti Powdered Monk Fruit Allulose Blend
- 2 tablespoon Unflavored gelatin powder
- 2 teaspoon Vanilla extract
- 1 cup Water
- 1/4 teaspoon Sea salt

Instructions

1. Use parchment paper to line an 8x8 inch baking pan. Set aside.
2. In a large mixing bowl, pour 1/2 cup warm water. Gelatin should be sprinkled over the water and whisked right away. Set aside.
3. In a large saucepan, combine the remaining 1/2 cup water, powdered sweetener, and sea salt. Heat for a few minutes over low to medium heat, often stirring, until the mixture is heated but not boiling and the sweetener has dissolved. As soon as bubbles begin to develop around the borders, the color will change from opaque to slightly translucent, and you should remove it quickly.
4. Remove the pan from the heat. Add the vanilla extract and mix well. While whisking regularly, pour the hot liquid into the big dish with the gelatin.
5. Beat the mixture for twelve-fifteen minutes on high speed with a hand mixer until the volume doubles and the mixture looks very bubbly, like stiff egg white peaks. The time will vary depending on the size of your bowl and the strength of your mixer.
6. Fill the prepared pan with the marshmallow mixture.
7. Refrigerate until solid and no longer sticky, at least 8 hours or overnight. Cut into squares using a sharp chef's knife.

LOW-CARB KETO BANANA MUFFINS

Prep Time: 10 Minutes

Cook Time: 20 Minutes

Serves: 10

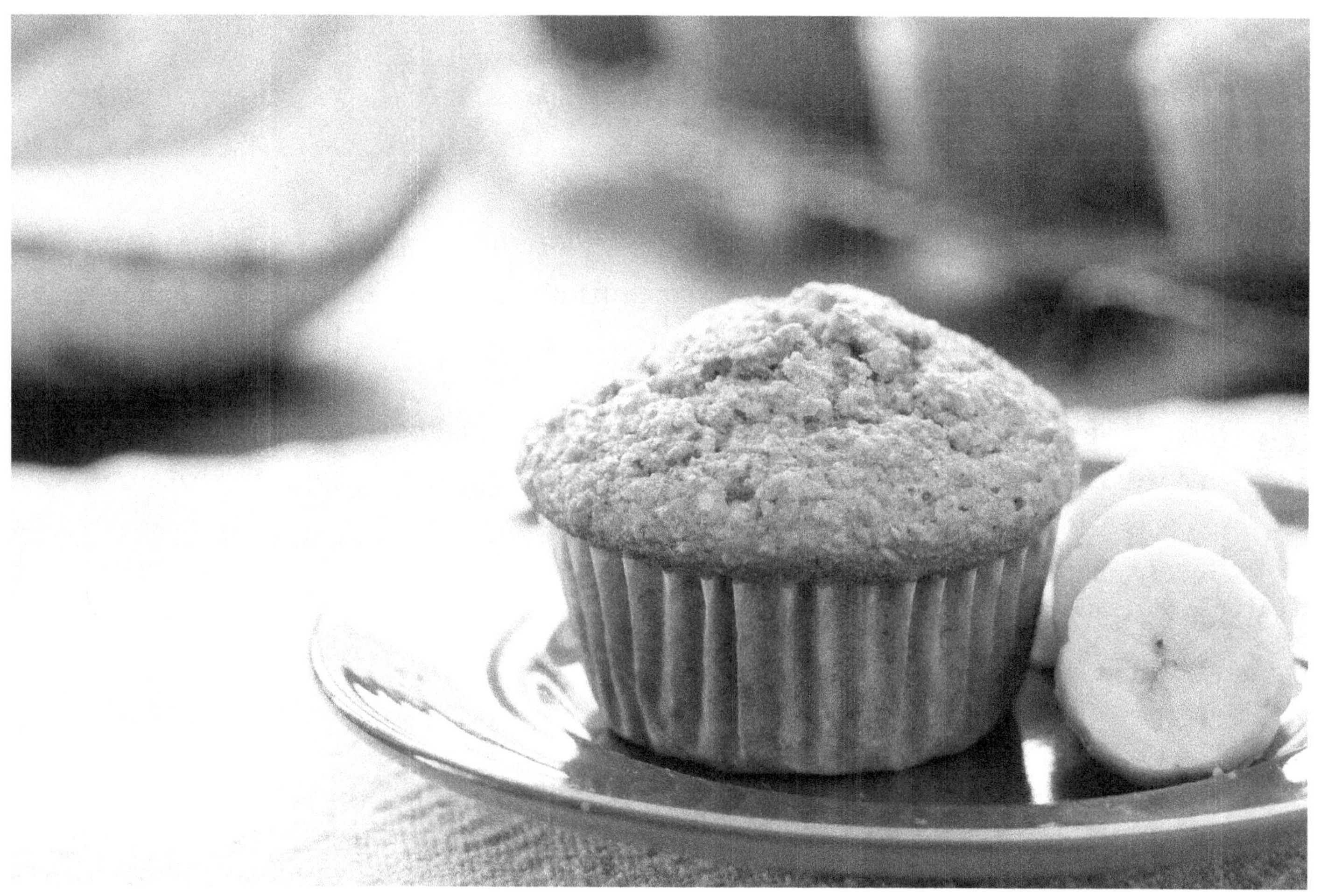

To fulfill your appetite, make these luscious, bakery-style keto banana muffins! A secret ingredient makes these sugar-free, low-carb banana muffins with almond flour taste just like banana bread without bananas.

Nutrition

Calories: 295 | Fat: 27.4g | Protein: 9.3g | Fiber: 3.6g | Sugar: 1.3g

Total Carbohydrates: 7.7g | Net Carbohydrates: 4.1g

Ingredients

- 3 large Eggs
- 2 1/2 cups Wholesome Yum Blanched Almond Flour
- 1/3 cup unsweetened almond milk
- 1/2 cup Besti Allulose
- 1 1/2 teaspoon Baking powder
- 3/4 cup Walnuts chopped
- 1 teaspoon Banana extract
- 1/3 cup butter
- 1/4 teaspoon Sea salt

Instructions

1. Preheat the oven to 350°F. Use 10 silicone or parchment paper muffin liners to line a muffin tray. Use 12 muffin tops for a lower calorie/carb count or 10 for a bigger muffin top.
2. Mix the almond flour, allulose, baking powder, and sea salt in a large mixing dish.
3. In a large mixing bowl, combine the melted butter, almond milk, eggs, and banana extract. Add 1/2 cup chopped walnuts to the mixture.
4. Evenly distribute the batter amongst the muffin cups. Top with the remaining walnuts.
5. Bake for twenty-twenty five minutes, or until golden on top and a toothpick inserted in the center comes out clean.